VITAL
infor

T4-AKY-332

What you need to know
ABOUT

Hospitals

BY DIANE BARNET, R.N.

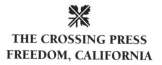

THE CROSSING PRESS
FREEDOM, CALIFORNIA

To WJB
and the
Old Quarry Group

The ideas, suggestions, and techniques in this book are not intended to be a substitute for professional health care. Anyone with a history of serious illness should consult a licensed practitioner.

For information on bulk purchases or group discounts for this and other Crossing Press titles, please contact our Special Sales Manager at 800-777-1048.

Visit our Web site on the Internet: www.crossingpress.com

Library of Congress Cataloging-in-Publication Data

Barnet, Diane.
     Hospitals / by Diane Barnet.
         p. cm. -- (Vital information series)
     Includes bibliographical references and index.
     ISBN 0-89594-908-3 (pbk.)
     1. Hospitals--Popular works. I. Title. II. Series.
RA963.B37   1998
362.1'1--dc21   98-26924
                                                        CIP

Contents

INTRODUCTION: Understanding the
Hospital Bureaucracy 5

PART I: UNDERSTANDING HOSPITALS: THE SYSTEMS AND THE PEOPLE

CHAPTER 1: HOSPITALS: Not Quite the Ritz 9

CHAPTER 2: ADMINISTRATION: The Buck Stops Here....23

CHAPTER 3: DOCTORS: Only Human 27

CHAPTER 4: NURSES: Florence Nightingale,
Where Are You? 36

CHAPTER 5: OTHER HOSPITAL WORKERS:
Who Did You Say You Were? 44

CHAPTER 6: PATIENTS: Special Issues to Consider 50

CHAPTER 7: PAYMENT: No Free Lunch 57

PART II: UNDERSTANDING TECHNICAL MATTERS

CHAPTER 8: BASIC BODY SYSTEMS: A Short Review.....62

CHAPTER 9: MEDICAL EQUIPMENT AND
PROCEDURES: A User-Friendly Guide.........71

CHAPTER 10: DRUGS: What You Don't Know
Can Hurt You 99

PART III: NEXT STEPS

CHAPTER 11: ON LEAVING THE HOSPITAL:
No Place Like Home 114

BIBLIOGRAPHY 121

INDEX 122

Introduction:
UNDERSTANDING THE
HOSPITAL BUREAUCRACY

AN OVERWHELMING EXPERIENCE

Sooner or later you will enter a hospital, either as a patient or a concerned visitor. But hospitals can be impersonal and confusing. Fear, joy, anxiety, relief, anger, frustration, and suspense—no other institution offers such a spectrum of intense birth-to-death emotions. Hospitals can intimidate everyone—even those people who are competent and in control in other areas of their lives.

The hospital fulfills many functions: It is part charity, part business, even part hotel on occasion. But consumer expectations of what it can provide are often unrealistic, fed by the media, the insurance companies, and, in some cases, the hospitals themselves. The public lacks accurate information about what hospitals do and how they work. And asking the wrong people can exacerbate problems. The overwhelming issue for patients and families is how best you can assert yourself in the unfamiliar hospital setting. How can you ensure that you or your loved one gets the best possible care?

SURVIVING THE HOSPITAL EXPERIENCE

The most successful patients are those who understand the idiosyncrasies of the hospital system and are not afraid to ask questions when there is something that they don't understand. The rise of the patient advocate or ombudsman indicates a growing recognition that reasonable questions have gone unanswered too often, to the detriment of hospitals' reputations and the well-being of those receiving care. It takes courage to question a hierarchy where employees, as well as clients, are conditioned to follow orders. Who wants to alienate the staff and risk experiencing resentment at a time when you are most vulnerable?

Today more and more consumers are taking steps to become fully informed partners in their medical treatment. Learning how hospitals work is essential in obtaining good health care. It involves taking some responsibility. You might be a patient one day. Unless you know the rules of the game and its key players, you might get lost in the shuffle.

Everyone has questions about hospitals:

▲ How can I make the system work for me or my loved ones?

▲ Why are hospitals so bureaucratically structured?

▲ Are there significant differences among them?

▲ Who is this doctor I've never seen before?

▲ Why do I have a different nurse every day?

▲ Where can I get more information? How can I check credentials?

If you have questions like these, then this book is essential reading for you. Unlike other books about hospitals and the health care system, it contains valuable insider tips, insights, and advice relevant to today's rapidly changing health care scene. It discusses special patient issues, methods of payment, and the transition from hospital to home. In addition, it provides lists for further reading and important organizations to contact for more information.

Also, here is a basic review of body systems and (I hope) a readable introduction to the medical equipment and frequently prescribed drugs you may encounter.

I hope this will help you weigh the facts, make decisions, and access the information you need in order to deal with hospitals as a well-informed consumer.

PART I
Understanding Hospitals:
THE SYSTEMS AND THE PEOPLE

CHAPTER 1: HOSPITALS: Not Quite the Ritz.....................9
  Types of Hospitals...9
  Hospital Inspections 11
  Hospital Costs 12
  Admission 13
  Hospital Amenities 17
  Visiting Hours..19
  Family Accommodations..19
  How a Hospital Unit Is Structured 19
  Discharge from the Hospital 21
  Getting VIP Treatment 21

CHAPTER 2: ADMINISTRATION: The Buck Stops Here.....23
  The Administration's Responsibilities 23
  Ensuring Quality Care...24
  Upholding Patient Rights 25
  Your Medical Record..25

CHAPTER 3: DOCTORS: Only Human 27
  Choosing a Doctor..27
  Talking with Your Doctor 28
  The Teaching Hospital Hierarchy 29
  Advantages of a Teaching Hospital 32
  Supervision of Physicians..32
  Qualities of a Good Doctor 33

**CHAPTER 4: NURSES: Florence Nightingale,
            Where Are You?**...36
  Who's Who in the Nursing Hierarchy..........................37
  A Changing Field 39
  Nursing Responsibilities..40
  Staffing Levels..41
  Unlicensed Staff 42
  Your Role..42
  Qualities of a Good Nurse 43

CHAPTER 5: OTHER HOSPITAL WORKERS:
                Who Did You Say You Were? 44
        Clerks..44
        Laboratory Technicians 44
        Imaging Technicians...45
        EKG Technicians 45
        Pharmacy Staff...45
        Health Educators 46
        Infection Control..46
        Rehabilitation Specialists..46
        Social Workers..47
        Pastoral Care Staff...47
        Mental Health Staff..48
        Patient Representatives..48
        Other Hospital Staff...49

CHAPTER 6: PATIENTS: Special Issues to Consider 50
        Advance Directive 50
        Visiting Policies..51
        Holistic Therapies..52
        What Makes a Good Patient? 53
        What Makes a Good Supporter?...................................54

CHAPTER 7: PAYMENT: No Free Lunch...........................57
        "Scholarship" Patients..57
        Hospital Billing Practices...58
        Reducing Hospital Costs 59

Hospitals:
NOT QUITE THE RITZ

There are hospitals and then there are hospitals. All are not created equal. They range from the Mayo Clinic, a world-famous, multibuilding medical complex, to small facilities in remote locations. Some have state-of-the-art trauma units. Others do not even have emergency rooms. Given this diversity in service, it is important to know what your local hospital offers.

TYPES OF HOSPITALS

Hospitals began in medieval times as institutions organized by the church to care for the sick and dying. Today's hospitals fall into a number of categories. They can be classified according to how they are financed:

- ▲ Not for profit
- ▲ For profit and frequently owned by large corporate chains
- ▲ Government funded

Hospitals can be either public or private, part charity, part business, or some combination of both. The result: a built-in conflict of roles for hospitals in our society. Hospitals are also categorized according to what they do:

- ▲ Community hospitals
- ▲ Teaching hospitals
- ▲ Specialty hospitals
- ▲ Rehabilitation hospitals
- ▲ Veterans Administration hospitals
- ▲ Government-run hospitals, including city, county, and state hospitals

COMMUNITY HOSPITALS

Community hospitals provide general medical services. They are staffed by attending physicians who are not direct employees of the hospitals, but have admitting privileges and refer their patients there. These doctors use the hospital facilities and are paid by patients through their insurers. Some community hospitals have chiefs of staff or department heads, who are paid directly by the hospital.

Community hospitals are usually adequate for routine procedures such as appendectomies, hip replacements, and gallbladder surgery. But teaching hospitals and major medical centers are more likely to offer burn units, infertility clinics, and transplant surgery. A community hospital may be adequate for treatment of a stroke, but if you have a brain tumor you will probably benefit more from a major teaching hospital's neurologists and neurosurgeons.

TEACHING HOSPITALS

Teaching hospitals are affiliated with university medical schools. They are the most prestigious in the hospital pecking order and frequently offer more specialized treatment than community hospitals. Their attending physicians supervise residents in various specialties and also function as professors in the medical school. Chapter Three details the medical hierarchy in teaching hospitals. Some community hospitals serve as teaching hospitals, but teaching facilities are more often larger city hospitals or hospitals connected to major medical centers.

ACUTE AND CHRONIC CARE

Acute care hospitals treat medical conditions that arise suddenly and are stabilized within a short time period. Examples include accidents, emergencies, and surgery. Chronic care hospitals treat patients who are in stable condition after a medical crisis has passed but who need further treatment to maintain their current status or gradually improve it. A patient who requires ongoing physical therapy after a stroke would be treated in a chronic care hospital.

GOVERNMENT HOSPITALS

City and county hospitals are frequently older, more crowded, and not so well funded as the more suburban community hospitals. They often began as charitable institutions. State hospitals most often treat mental illness of a long-term or chronic nature. Veterans Administration hospitals treat Armed Forces veterans.

SPECIALTY HOSPITALS

Specialty hospitals focus on specific diseases or conditions. They include:

▲ Orthopedic hospitals that treat bone problems

▲ Cancer treatment centers

▲ Private psychiatric hospitals

▲ Rehabilitation and convalescent hospitals that treat patients who are past the acute stage of their injury or illness but who require ongoing care

OVERLAPPING CATEGORIES

The picture is further muddied when we try to describe hospitals according to how they are funded and see that the various categories overlap. Community hospitals may be either not-for-profit or for-profit facilities. Teaching hospitals may be either city, county, state, VA, or community hospitals. There are also church-affiliated hospitals that function as general hospitals. Some have special restrictions. For instance, a Seventh–day Adventist hospital might adhere to that church's dietary laws and not serve drinks containing caffeine.

HOSPITAL INSPECTIONS

Hospitals are inspected every three years by the Joint Commission on Accreditation of Healthcare Organizations (JCAHO). This is a private organization started by doctors and hospitals themselves to ensure that hospitals meet certain minimal standards. In a given year, 80 percent of hospitals pass their inspections. The scores the hospitals received in the inspection of their sites are public knowledge and can be obtained by contacting the JCAHO. (The address is listed at the back of this book.)

HOSPITAL COSTS

Hospital bills include what are called the "usual and customary" charges for the hospital room. These room charges include meals, housekeeping, and nursing services. Other charges for drugs, equipment used, tests, etc. are itemized separately. There may be additional charges for such extras as cable TV and phone calls.

The largest group of patients—up to 50 percent in some hospitals—are eligible for Medicare. The federal Health Care Financing Administration (HCFA) oversees Medicare. In 1983, hospitals began to be reimbursed in fixed amounts based on the diagnosis for care given to Medicare patients. A list of over 400 illnesses was established and organized into Diagnostic Related Groupings (DRGs). There is a predetermined length of stay and ceiling amount paid to hospitals for the treatment of each DRG.

However, the fees Medicare pays for treatment are 30 percent to 50 percent lower than most doctors' fees. As a result, some doctors do not "accept assignment" or take on any new Medicare patients. For non-Medicare patients, insurance companies also have limits on how long patients may stay and how much they will pay for any given illness. All these factors affect the rates hospitals charge.

The cost of your hospital room is as high as it is because while you may stay only three of the average four days that your insurer allows for your surgery, Mrs. Jones may have the same operation, develop complications, and stay ten days. In addition, even for-profit hospitals often accept a few patients who do not have insurance as "charity" or "scholarship" patients. An uninsured youth injured in a motorcycle accident fits this description. As a result, insured patients indirectly pick up the tab. Hospitals get revenue in other ways, too, such as charging high markups on everything from rooms to boxes of tissues. See Chapter Three for further discussion of your hospital bill.

ADMISSION

Admission to the hospital is either **elective** (preplanned) or emergency.

EMERGENCIES

Your first contact with the hospital may be the emergency room (**ER**). By law ERs cannot deny treatment. In some cities, certain ERs may at times have to stop accepting cases if they become too full. Emergency ambulance services must then divert to other hospitals. Unfortunately, too often the public abuses ERs by going there for minor problems, which clogs the system. Sorting out patients according to the severity of their symptoms, called "triage," is usually done by a nurse. But in some ERs, a clerical employee without medical or nursing training makes these initial decisions. Some ER doctors are specialists in emergency medicine. Others are merely moonlighting and have no specialized training in this area.

CHOOSING A HOSPITAL

Apart from emergencies over which you have no control, where you go for hospitalization depends on where your doctor has admitting privileges. If he or she admits patients to more than one hospital, discuss the choices. Another factor that influences where you go is whether your insurance will pay for hospitalization in a particular facility. This is a concern in managed care. Frequently a managed care plan uses a specific network of hospitals. You pay more if you go outside the network.

QUESTIONS TO ASK UPON ADMISSION

▲ *Do I have all the patient information booklets, brochures, and information the hospital provides, including a "Patients' Bill of Rights"?*

▲ *What is included in any general consent form I sign? (Usually a general consent form describes admission, general treatment, lab tests, and X-rays. Consent forms for surgery and other medical procedures are discussed and explained later by physicians. Signatures are usually witnessed by nurses.)*

▲ *Do I understand all financial arrangements, including insurance coverage, acceptance of deposits, and credit arrangements?*

▲ *What is my room assignment and can it be changed if unacceptable?*

▲ *Will I be charged for TV whether or not I watch it?*

▲ *Can I rent or bring a VCR from home if I want to watch videos?*

▲ *What are the hospital visiting hours?*

▲ *What are the parking arrangements for visitors?*

▲ *Do I have information on how to contact the patient representative, chaplain, and social services department?*

If you are being treated by a specialist, you may be admitted to a hospital in a distant city. The disruption this causes can be a worthwhile trade-off for expert treatment. For instance, Jack, a sixty-year-old engineer, was suddenly diagnosed with bladder cancer. Fortunately, his insurance did not limit his choices geographically. He considered treatment at his two local general hospitals and at a major cancer center three hours' drive away. The local hospitals offered standard treatment, which involved removal of the tumor, chemotherapy, and the construction of an ileostomy, in which the bladder opens directly into a small, removable bag. Jack opted for treatment at the cancer center where, in a state-of-the-art procedure, a surgeon was able to construct a new bladder.

MANAGED CARE

A managed care organization groups a number of hospitals and doctors into a network to deliver care more efficiently to the patients who are enrolled in a managed care plan. One advantage is lower costs through controlling inappropriate overuse of medical services and buying equipment and supplies in bulk. A disadvantage is that you pay more for care if you seek it outside the network. Managed care networks vary in size and are organized in various ways. The most common varieties are Health Maintenance Organizations (HMOs) and Preferred Provider Organizations (PPOs). The majority of patients who are insured through their employers are now enrolled in some form of managed care.

THE ADMISSION PROCESS

Most insurers require precertification for **elective** (nonemergency) surgery at least forty-eight hours ahead of time. But even if you have an emergency admission, you should inform your insurer within twenty-four hours. For elective admissions, your doctor will send the hospital a preadmission form. Precertification by your insurer is needed and gives you a certification or approval number. You pass this on to your doctor's office or the hospital for their information.

The hospital admitting office usually calls you to reconfirm the day you're scheduled for admission. You can also call them to check. Some send a preadmission form or ask you to come to the hospital a few weeks ahead to fill out all admission paperwork. But beware: For elective admissions it is always possible that you may be "bumped" from the schedule and your admission postponed to a later date.

Early afternoon is the preferred check-in time. Most discharged patients leave by noon, but rooms may not be cleaned and ready until midafternoon. Often, these days, you'll arrive at the hospital on the morning of your surgery, having had pre-surgery tests as an outpatient. And some surgery is now done on an outpatient or day-surgery basis.

WHAT TO TAKE TO THE HOSPITAL

▲ *Health insurance cards*

▲ *Writing pad and pens*

▲ *Watch or small clock*

▲ *Basic toiletries*

▲ *Phone numbers of family and friends (tape them to your bedside table)*

▲ *Reading material*

▲ *Slippers with flat, nonslip soles and a robe that's easy to get in and out of, that preferably opens all the way down the front*

▲ *Nightgown/pajamas that have loose sleeves (tight sleeves are difficult if you have an IV—it's easier just to wear a hospital gown)*

▲ *Headphones and tapes/small radio (avoid bringing expensive items)*

▲ *Ear plugs/sleeping mask*

▲ *Any small item of spiritual or morale-building importance, such as a picture, religious item, or stuffed mascot*

▲ *Electric razor/hair drier: many units have these for patients' use (if you bring your own, maintenance will check them to ensure they're functioning properly and not a safety hazard)*

DO NOT BRING...

▲ *Credit cards or cash over a few dollars*

▲ *Jewelry*

▲ *Food, alcohol, or nonprescription drugs (if you bring prescribed drugs, give them to a nurse for safe-keeping)*

▲ *Large amounts of clothing/luggage*

Upon admission, you will be asked to provide insurance information if you haven't already done so. If uninsured, one alternative is to pay a deposit and have the patient accounts office work out a payment schedule. In addition, you should also get a patient information handbook, a copy of the hospital's Patients' Bill of Rights (see page 18), and information about an advance directive. Advance directive forms can be obtained at any time from doctors' and attorneys' offices, and it is a good idea to have one or more copies filed in a safe place well in advance of any hospital admission. You don't need an attorney to do these.

HOSPITAL AMENITIES

While being admitted and given a plastic bracelet with an identification number, you have a chance to look around you. A hospital's appearance has little to do with the quality of care. Don't be seduced by an attractive color scheme. Decor alone doesn't do it! There are community hospitals with marble lobbies, exotic plants, and piped-in music that deliver mediocre care at best. There are dark and decrepit city hospitals affiliated with medical schools where the care is excellent. Are you there for the view or the best treatment? Other hospital amenities such as comfortable waiting rooms, gift shops, and cafeterias are nice, but have no relation to medical care.

ROOMS

You may not get a private room even though your insurance covers it. Private rooms are often available only on a first-come, first-served basis and are sometimes unavailable. You will be given a semiprivate room and moved to a private room as soon as one is ready. On the other hand, if you have only semiprivate coverage but these beds are filled, you'll be given a private room temporarily but not charged for it. Conversely, sometimes you may get a private room for medical reasons, such as a serious infection that requires isolation for your own protection and for the protection of others.

PATIENTS' BILL OF RIGHTS

1. *The patient has a right to considerate and respectful care.*

2. *The patient has the right to obtain from physicians and other direct caregivers relevant, current, and understandable information concerning diagnosis, treatment, and prognosis.*

3. *The patient has the right to make decisions about the plan of care prior to and during the course of treatment and to refuse care.*

4. *The patient has the right to have an advance directive (such as a living will, health care proxy, or durable power of attorney for health care).*

5. *The patient has the right to every consideration of privacy.*

6. *The patient has the right to expect that all communications and records pertaining to his/her care will be treated as confidential by the hospital.*

7. *The patient has the right to review the records pertaining to his/her medical care.*

8. *The patient has the right to expect that the hospital will give appropriate and medically indicated care and services.*

9. *The patient has the right to be told of any business relationships among the hospital and other care providers, payers, or educational institutions that may influence treatment and care.*

10. *The patient has the right to refuse to participate in any research studies or human experimentation affecting care and treatment.*

11. *The patient has the right to expect reasonable continuity of care and to be offered further options when hospital care is no longer appropriate.*

12. *The patient has the right to be informed of hospital policies and practices that relate to patient care and of available resources for resolving disputes, as well as to be informed of the hospital's charges for services and available payment methods.*

HOSPITAL FOOD

Hospital food is often cause for complaint. Menus offer two or three choices for each meal and are filled out a day ahead. This means that you take "pot luck" the first day. You can request foods not listed on the menu, provided they are compatible with any special diet prescribed for you. Even so, it's not quite like home. But look at it this way: If you have a hearty appetite or can complain about the meals, you're probably not very sick! In many countries, patients do not have menu choices at all, but must accept what they're given or rely on family members to supply meals.

VISITING HOURS

Visiting policies vary. Many hospitals allow unlimited visiting in private rooms. They may provide a cot or folding bed for a family member who wishes to stay overnight with you. Visiting hours for semiprivate rooms are usually from 11:00 A.M. to 8:30 P.M.

FAMILY ACCOMMODATIONS

When you are hospitalized in a distant city, there is often nearby housing provided for visiting family. The best known are the Ronald McDonald houses for the families of children being treated away from home. Information on inexpensive accommodations for visitors can be obtained from the hospital admitting office, social services department, or pastoral care office.

HOW A HOSPITAL UNIT IS STRUCTURED

Each hospital floor, ward, or unit has its own routines and pecking order. Head nurses, sometimes called unit managers, are usually responsible for all activities on the units. They usually work only weekdays. However, at all times one nurse is designated as "in charge." Called the "charge nurse," this nurse is responsible for running the unit during the shift. The charge nurse does not usually take care of patients, but does administrative work at the nurses' station and helps out when needed. Direct any medical questions your nurse can't answer to the charge nurse.

A unit clerk, who is not a nurse, answers phones at the nurses' station and assists with clerical tasks and the high volume of paperwork hospitals generate. Nonmedical questions—about parking or visiting hours, for instance—the unit clerk can answer. This saves time for the nurses. The unit clerk can also call maintenance to fix the light in your room or tell you where the kitchenette is, for instance.

Hospital staffing shifts are usually either eight or twelve hours. For eight-hour shifts, days are from 7:00 A.M. to 3:00 P.M., evenings from 3:00 P.M. to 11:00 P.M., and nights from 11:00 P.M. to 7:00 A.M. Twelve-hour shifts run from 7:00 A.M. to 7:00 P.M. or vice versa. Military time is used in hospital charting and records, so that 1:00 P.M. is referred to as 1300 hours. Nurses who work twelve-hour shifts most often do no more than three in succession and then have three or four days off. Many hospitals have eight-hour shifts Monday through Friday and twelve-hour shifts over the weekend. The weekend staff may be totally different from the weekday staff.

There is a predictable pattern to hospital shifts. Toward the end of each shift, the charge nurse gets either a written or verbal report from every nurse about their patients. Before going off duty, the charge nurse then gives a taped or verbal report to the on-coming charge nurse, who will take over and assign patients to the new staff. Each on-coming nurse pairs up with the nurse whose patients she/he will take over for a one-on-one update. This is called the change-of-shift report. As a patient, you can find out when this occurs and avoid calling the nurse during a forty-five-minute period around this time. It is a busy time, with fewer staff available on the floor, and it will take longer to get a response.

The most common staffing pattern is to assign each nurse several patients. On a thirty-six-bed unit with six nurses, each nurse would have six patients. Some units use a team approach, where two team leaders each look after half the unit, supervising a number of nurses and aides, but reporting ultimately to the charge nurse. Another approach is primary nursing. Here, the nurse who first takes care of you upon admission writes a nursing care plan for you and coordinates your care, though the nurse will look after you directly only during her/his own shifts

Many units have a blackboard or greaseboard near the nurses' station that lists room numbers. Patients' names are entered on it along with the names of nurses assigned to the patients each shift. The first nurse you stop in a corridor may know only her/his own patients. It's wise to consult this board, the unit clerk, or the charge nurse to locate a patient's nurse for an update on the patient's condition. Your wife, for instance, might be in room 416, but there isn't a nurse in sight. This is because her nurse for this shift, Karen, has the patients in rooms 412 through 420 and happens to be in room 414 at the moment.

In many hospitals, a nurse or aide entering a room presses a wall button to activate a light outside the room over the door. This indicates a staff member is inside. You will also have a call button that causes the light outside the door to blink, as well as show up on a board at the nurses' station, alerting staff that you need help. There is often an intercom speaking system between each room and the nurses' station. The staff sometimes wear pagers as well.

DISCHARGE FROM THE HOSPITAL

You may be discharged earlier than expected if you are doing well. Most patients are happy to go home. But if you feel you are being discharged too soon, talk to your doctor. If your length of stay is based on the rules set by your insurer, your doctor can intervene and talk to them. There is also an appeal procedure for Medicare patients. Ask to speak to a nursing supervisor, hospital administrator, the social services department, or patient advocate. Many hospitals have a utilization review process that reviews patients' charts to monitor and track patient flow. Specially trained nurses read the charts and can speed treatment along by recommending discharge if they feel the patient is ready. You are always free to leave at any time, but must sign a release to show that you left "against medical advice" (AMA) if the doctor has not written a discharge order.

GETTING VIP TREATMENT

Most community hospitals and major medical centers have public relations and even marketing departments. They tend to give VIP treatment to patients they consider to be important members of the community. So if your wife is a city councilor, your brother a doctor (never mind that he lives in Alaska), or your son a nurse, mention it. You may get extra attention if it is felt that you have extra clout in the community or know more than the average patient. This sounds unfair and unethical. After all, shouldn't every patient get VIP treatment? But this is how hospitals work.

Hospitals are unfamiliar environments and are undeniably stressful for you as a patient, as well as for your family and friends. Some of this stress is due to your lack of information and control over your situation. But by the time you finish this book, you will know more than you did before and will be better equipped to ask knowledgeable questions about the system.

Administration:
THE BUCK STOPS HERE

Each hospital's administration is unique. An administrator's job is to run the hospital efficiently and preserve its public image. Administrators manage money, personnel, and materials. They make decisions, hire and fire, take the heat, and get the credit. The administrator is hired by, and reports to, the hospital's board of trustees, directors, or governors. The administrator is also sometimes the Chief Executive Officer (CEO). She/he may be a voting member of the board, though never the chairperson. The administrator and the board function as partners and are ultimately responsible for the care of the patents who are admitted.

THE ADMINISTRATOR'S RESPONSIBILITIES

An administrator deals with both internal and community aspects of hospital management. Within the hospital she/he:

▲ Keep the staff informed of organizational changes, board decisions, and anything else that affects them

▲ Establishes and reviews hospital policies

▲ Recruits and retains staff and is answerable for their actions

▲ Supervises the day-to-day running of the facility, including maintenance and construction

▲ Prepares monthly financial statements and annual budgets for approval by the board

▲ Negotiates reimbursements from third-party insurers

The administrator's activities in the community are numerous. They include:

▲ Maintaining good community relations

▲ Producing publications such as newsletters and press releases

▲ Presenting a positive image of the hospital

The administrator must handle complaints from patients and families and must also be aware of the constantly changing government regulations related to funding, reimbursement, and planning.

There may be one or more assistant administrators responsible for specific areas such as plant operations. Various departments take care of the acquisition and management of capital, accounting, payroll, patient accounts, human resources, employee health, medical records, nursing, social work, public relations, and marketing. All these departments affect patient care directly or indirectly.

ENSURING QUALITY CARE

Litigation and negative media exposure are the administration's twin terrors. Most hospitals now have a quality assurance program in effect to prevent these from occurring. Quality assurance usually consists of such components as a utilization review department and a medical audit committee. Utilization review is simply a system set up to review the necessity, quality, and appropriateness of care provided during each patient's hospitalization. It attempts to monitor treatment from first admission throughout the length of stay and discharge planning. A utilization review committee works with such entities as a medical records committee and a medical audit committee to review clinical practice in the hospital.

A medical audit system is how the medical staff tracks its own activities. It may include:

▲ A credentials committee to monitor doctors' qualifications

▲ A tissue committee that determines through tests whether surgery is necessary

▲ A medicolegal committee to deal with legal and ethical issues

▲ A mortality and morbidity committee to review statistics on hospital deaths and illnesses

Quality assurance interacts with the hospital's risk management team. Both help prevent malpractice suits, but while quality assurance is set up to help patients, risk management helps protect the hospital's assets. It involves receiving, maintaining, and evaluating reports on accidents and other incidents that occur in the hospital. It looks for possible causes of liability. A risk management team may include some of the administrative staff, the board of directors, doctors, other employees, an attorney for the hospital, and insurance consultants.

UPHOLDING PATIENT RIGHTS

In addition, the American Hospital Association has adopted a standard Code of Patients' Rights that hospitals voluntarily observe (see page 18). The code is usually posted in a prominent place and each patient receives a copy on admission. There are a dozen basic rights listed. They include the right to:

▲ Receive respectful care

▲ Obtain information

▲ Make decisions

You can take certain steps to safeguard your rights. For instance, you can revise or amend consent forms to state that you refuse to let anyone but your own doctor perform surgery. You can also withdraw consent at any time.

YOUR MEDICAL RECORD

There are a number of reasons why you may want to keep copies of your medical records. Your medical history is important background information that your doctors need to know when considering any future treatment, even if it's years down the road. When seeking a second opinion, you need your records. In the case of any insurance or legal dispute, it's also an advantage to have your own records. Records kept in doctors' offices and hospitals are sometimes lost or misplaced, and some hospitals destroy certain records, such as X-rays, after several years. Having your own copies may also prevent unnecessary and costly duplication of X-rays and tests.

In most states, you have the right to see and copy your medical records. Technically, the actual files belong to the hospital, but the information belongs to you. In some states, you may be required to pay for copying costs, or you may have access only after leaving the hospital or only to some portions of your chart, such as X-rays and lab reports. In other states, you may be entitled only to a summary of your chart or may have to show good cause as to why you need your records. After two or three years, most medical records are transferred to microfilm for storage.

Approach your doctor, a patient representative, or the administrator if you want to see your chart. You may also make a formal request through an attorney, if necessary. If denied access you have a right to appeal to your state health department.

Your medical chart's discharge summary is in many ways the most important section because it includes a discussion of your condition at the time of dismissal from the hospital as well as recommendations for future treatment.

Bear in mind that you may need someone with a medical or nursing background to help you interpret some of the information or put it into proper perspective. If you don't know any nurses, doctors, or medical or nursing students, there are businesses called "cost review" or "medical review" companies who can help you.

As a patient, you could probably have a satisfactory hospital experience without ever being aware of any of the material in this chapter. Much of it is behind-the-scenes information that the average patient doesn't need to know unless a problem occurs. But a smoothly functioning administration is crucial to the delivery of quality care. And part of the hospital's responsibility is to protect your rights as a patient.

Doctors:
ONLY HUMAN

Many people choose their hairstylists or mechanics more carefully than they choose their doctors. While it can be reassuring to have a primary care doctor you trust and who makes you feel comfortable, bedside manner alone is of limited value. A "feel good" doctor may be a mediocre diagnostician or surgeon, while a doctor who communicates poorly may be a good clinician. In fact, it may be unrealistic to expect a doctor to be both warmly personable and a clinical expert. Doctors are not gods; they are only human.

CHOOSING A DOCTOR

You probably go to a family practitioner or internist as a first response when you need care. These doctors deal mostly with routine conditions; unusual or serious problems require referral to a specialist. If your doctor refers you to a specialist, you can check the specialist's credentials with the state licensing board or board of registration. These agencies ensure that an individual has at least the minimum qualifications for the job. Specialists should have passed examinations held under the jurisdiction of special boards, such as the American Board of Surgery, as a minimal standard of practice in a specialty. Board certification requirements also include that a specialist stay in active practice and keep up with developments in the specialty through continuing education credits.

Managed care plans, such as Health Maintenance Organizations (HMOs), limit patients to doctors within specific networks of health care providers. Some have very short lists of specialists. This can be cause for concern, as it may reduce the level of expertise available to you. For example, suppose you have an infant who needs corrective bladder surgery. You belong to an HMO that lists five urologists, none of whom specializes in pediatric urology. Your dilemma is whether to stay within the network and go to a urologist who does only a few such procedures a year, or pay more to seek a pediatric urologist who is outside the HMO but does hundreds of these operations. Leaving an HMO network's list of health care providers usually costs more. When considering surgery, it is important to get a second, or even third, opinion. Many HMOs and other insurers require a second opinion.

Nurses are often the best source of inside information on doctors, especially if a nurse has worked in the same hospital or specialty area for many years. Nurses see patients who have been treated by specific doctors, and they often gain an objective overview of each doctor's competence. Nurses can answer the following questions:

▲ Does the doctor care deeply about his or her patients?

▲ Does he return calls?

▲ Is she open to suggestion?

▲ Is he thorough?

▲ What is her rate of complications?

If you don't know any nurses and are facing surgery, one approach is to call the operating room suite and ask the nurse in charge, who can remain anonymous, to recommend a good surgeon. You can also request a specific anesthesiologist.

TALKING WITH YOUR DOCTOR

Your relationship with your doctor should be one of equals. Some doctors are better at communicating than others, however. Whether yours is easy to talk to or not, organize your questions ahead of time and look up as much information as possible on your own. Many bookstores and public libraries have medical sections with books for the lay person on every conceivable disease or condition, and there are Internet resources with health information as well. Always ask questions. Here are some basics:

▲ Is this treatment/procedure necessary?

▲ What are the alternatives?

▲ What are the potential complications?

▲ Will I be hospitalized? If so, for how long?

▲ How long will my recovery period last?

The most useful open-ended question is simply, "What are the implications?"

Communication with your doctor is a two-way street. Doctors usually appreciate a well-informed patient. You are responsible for providing clear, concise, and specific information, if at all possible. Too many patients feel that their doctors can somehow read their minds. The more detailed and specific the information you provide, the better picture your doctor will have to work with. A patient who provides clear information as to his or her medical history and symptoms is called a "good historian" in medical parlance. A "poor historian" gives vague answers and fuzzy, contradictory information. Doctors find this frustrating. Hiding facts due to embarrassment should be avoided; doctors have heard it all before. Discussion of all possible outcomes can ensure that your expectations are realistic and can prevent later misunderstanding. The consent forms required by most hospitals call for "informed" consent, after all, and can be amended or altered.

THE TEACHING HOSPITAL HIERARCHY

In community hospitals, doctors are not direct employees of the hospital but have admitting privileges and are called "attending physicians." Teaching hospitals, affiliated with medical schools, present a more complex hierarchy of doctors. At the bottom of the totem pole are fourth-year medical students, sometimes called "clinical clerks." Then come various categories of residents. Finally, there are the specialists, fully qualified doctors who also teach at the medical school.

MEDICAL STUDENTS

Most students spend their first two years of medical school in labs and classrooms, and only begin to see "real" patients during the last two years. At this stage in their training, they learn to diagnose and treat patients, but are supervised by more experienced medical staff who must approve and countersign any orders students write for patients. Once a medical student has passed final qualifying exams, he or she can use the title MD, but the fledgling doctor's medical education has just begun. The term "intern" is now almost obsolete. Years ago, an internship was a one-year rotation through several specialties, typically surgery, obstetrics, pediatrics, and psychiatry. After that year, a doctor either set up in family practice or embarked on a residency in a specialty. But today, medicine is so complex and the body of knowledge expanding so rapidly, with subspecialties within specialties, that most medical graduates go straight into residency programs. Even those who plan on family practice complete a residency of two years or more.

RESIDENTS

Residents are considered hospital employees. Residents put in long hours at low pay. They form the core medical service in teaching hospitals, especially on weekends and at night, while earning approximately the same salary as a unit nurse. Residencies can last up to seven years in some specialties. There are dozens of specialties, not just pediatrics or cardiology, for instance, but pediatric cardiology. There are also behind-the-scenes specialties such as pathology, radiology, and nuclear medicine, where doctors seldom see patients face-to-face. Residents are part of a pecking order that starts with the junior and senior residents and ascends to the chief resident. A first-year junior resident is often called a "PGY 1," which stands for "post-graduate year one." In a large teaching hospital, there may be several senior and junior residents in each specialty. Considerable differences in experience and skill exist between a chief resident, who is often at the peak of his or her ability after years of concentration in a specialty, and a new junior resident. But all of them work for and with fully qualified specialists.

As a patient, you can refuse to have any invasive procedure performed by a student or resident. Invasive procedures include anything that breaks the skin barrier—starting an intravenous line, drawing blood for tests, or doing a spinal tap to obtain cerebrospinal fluid, for instance. A resident could be doing it for the first time. In any case, there is an unofficial "three strikes, you're out" rule that you should keep in mind: If, after three attempts, an employee can't complete a procedure, it's time to request that someone else do it. For example, don't let anyone try more than three times to start an IV. Ask for a different person. Although there are some things only doctors are licensed to do, nurses often do better at some procedures, such as starting IVs. Some hospitals have an "IV Team" of nurses or technicians who specialize in starting IVs and drawing blood.

SPECIALISTS

In teaching hospitals, specialists make regular rounds to see patients, subject to the demands of emergencies, operating room schedules, and classroom lectures. Typically, the specialist sweeps into the patient's room followed by a parade of residents, students, and a nurse. No wonder you might feel like Exhibit A in a sideshow. But you also benefit from the medical team's collective attention. One of them may notice something, ask a question, or make a suggestion that others may not have considered.

While many specialists routinely perform surgery (gynecologists, obstetricians, and urologists, for instance), others do not (internists and endocrinologists, for example). Among surgeons, there are general surgeons and those who specialize. A cardiac surgeon would do only heart surgery, while a cardiologist diagnoses and treats heart problems by nonsurgical means, referring a patient to a cardiac surgeon when necessary. There are also behind-the-scenes specialists, such as radiologists, who study and interpret X-rays and other diagnostic tests. Pathologists study tissue removed during surgery.

Doctors should make their status clear. When Tom Brown took his child to the emergency room at his local university medical center teaching hospital, a resident appeared with a medical student in tow. "I'm Dr. Smith," he said, "and this is Dr. Klein." Maybe the resident assumed that Tom knew nothing about the hospital's hierarchy of doctors or that he would be uncomfortable with a student present. Perhaps he did not want to give a lengthy explanation of the fourth-year student's non-MD status. Nevertheless, this misrepresentation was unethical and somewhat patronizing.

ADVANTAGES OF A TEACHING HOSPITAL

An advantage of a teaching hospital is that residents are keen, thorough, and enthusiastic. There are more checks and balances at play when it comes to patient care, and more awareness of current research and treatment due to the medical school connection of teaching hospitals. A potential disadvantage is that a patient may, on occasion, feel like a guinea pig or teaching tool and may be subject to a trainee's inexperience.

Obviously no doctor can be on call and available twenty-four hours a day, every day. At community hospitals, doctors cover for each other on weekends and holidays. But in teaching hospitals, residents are on call in rotating shifts around the clock. If you, as a patient, develop a problem, you'll be seen first by a resident, usually not the top specialist. The amount of time a doctor can spend with you is often in inverse ratio to his or her seniority. A fourth-year medical student may take forty-five minutes to do a physical exam, take a medical history, and write copious notes on a new patient. This work will be checked by senior residents. The chief resident may spend only minutes with a patient. But in an emergency, a resident will be called to assess the situation quickly and notify a specialist, if necessary.

SUPERVISION OF PHYSICIANS

Hospitals are responsible for the actions of their doctors, even if a doctor is working for an outside agency that is under contract to the hospital. If you believe that a doctor has acted negligently or unethically, you can go to the hospital administrator with your concern. Hospitals have ethics committees whose mandate is to prevent and correct problems. You can also file a written complaint with the state licensing board, which may investigate and take action against a doctor.

Malpractice litigation sets out to prove that the doctor, who had a duty to provide you with a reasonable standard of care, breached that duty. Physical or mental harm must result from proven negligence, not mere misadventure. Expert medical witnesses and attorneys who specialize in this field are inevitably involved in any malpractice suit, which may take years to resolve or be settled out of court.

As a patient, you may encounter doctors who received their basic medical education in another country. Some may be Americans who studied medicine abroad in Europe, Mexico, or the Caribbean. Foreign-trained doctors may be as well qualified as American-trained doctors. Those educated in Canada, Europe, Australia, New Zealand, South Africa, and Israel are often at least as well qualified as Americans. Doctors from other areas of the world are often better equipped to meet American standards if they have completed residency programs or some form of advanced training in the United States. In a field like psychiatry, where sociocultural factors play a larger role than in, say, orthopedics, foreign-trained doctors may be problematic. If from a very different culture, a doctor can miss important clues when talking to you. In recent years, many state hospitals—which treat chronic mentally ill and developmentally handicapped patients—have had difficulty attracting psychiatrists. Many have hired large numbers of foreign-trained psychiatrists. Their cultural baggage, through no fault of their own, may impose barriers between doctor and patient.

The bottom line is not to take anything for granted. Don't assume anything, including that a doctor can read your mind. Find out as much as you can. Ask questions—lots of questions. This is no time for timidity. A middle-aged woman was about to be wheeled into surgery. As she waited in a holding area, she asked querulously, "Is the doctor a specialist?" Considering that her surgery had been scheduled weeks ago, the timing of her question was far from optimal.

QUALITIES OF A GOOD DOCTOR

What makes a good doctor? Obviously you expect the doctor to be competent and professional. Beyond this basic assumption, you probably want your doctor to be approachable, to listen to you, and treat you as an equal. A bored, dismissive, or patronizing attitude does not inspire trust, nor does a doctor who feels threatened by your questions. A good doctor will answer questions, but not be afraid to admit it when he or she doesn't know all the answers.

A good doctor will find out. A good doctor will welcome your wish for a second opinion.

A good doctor should not force ideas or treatment on you. She or he should treat you as an individual and explain treatment at a level you can understand. After all, you are a health care consumer who is employing the doctor. Susan was an active fifty-year-old woman who was sailing through menopause with very few problems. She visited a new doctor for a routine checkup. "Are you taking estrogen?" he asked.

"No," she replied, "I've thought about it and read everything I can about it, but nothing has convinced me that I need it, so far."

"I put most women patients your age on hormone replacement therapy," he said.

That was the last time Susan saw him. "I'm not 'most patients,'" she said. "I'm me, an individual." Happily, she found a new doctor who was willing to let her make up her own mind about this still somewhat-controversial treatment.

TYPES OF PHYSICIANS

MD   *Doctor of Medicine*

DO   *Doctor of Osteopathy, a medical system based on the theory that diseases are caused by an imbalance or loss of structural integrity in the body and can be cured by a manipulation of the parts, supplemented by other therapeutic measures.*

DC   *Doctor of Chiropractic, a system of treatment that involves manipulation of the backbone. This is thought to relieve pressure on the nerves so that the body can restore itself to health.*

DPM   *Doctor of Podiatry, diseases of the foot*

COMMON MEDICAL SPECIALISTS

SPECIALIST	AREA OF SPECIALIZATION
Cardiologist	*Heart problems*
Dermatologist	*Skin problems*
Endocrinologist	*Problems related to glands, hormones, and metabolism*
Gynecologist	*The female reproductive system*
Internist	*Problems in the body's major organs*
Hematologist	*Diseases of the blood*
Nephrologist	*Kidney problems*
Neurologist	*Disorders of the nervous system*
Oncologist	*Cancer specialist*
Ophthalmologist	*Eye diseases*
Orthopedist	*Bone problems*
Obstetrician	*Childbirth*
Pediatrician	*Children's health*
Psychiatrist	*Treatment of mental and emotional disorders*
Rheumatologist	*Diseases of the joints, muscles, and immune system*
Urologist	*Diseases of the bladder and urinary system*

Nurses:

FLORENCE NIGHTINGALE, WHERE ARE YOU?

Y ou are a patient. You are talking on the phone when a nurse you've never seen before enters your room with a small plastic cup of pills. "Just leave them on the table," you say, returning to your conversation.

"No, I'll come back," she answers and starts to leave with the pills in her hand.

"It's all right," you protest, "I really will take them."

"I'm not allowed to leave them; it's hospital policy," is her response.

Feeling vaguely insulted—after all, you are a responsible grown-up—you resignedly interrupt your call to swallow the pills on the spot with the nurse as witness.

Ideally, you and the nurse are a team. In this case, the nurse's actions were correct, as was the medication. When a nurse brings your medication, it's your right to ask questions. A good nurse will not resent this since it also protects him or her. Although bringing the correct medication was not the issue here, mistakes happen. The nurse should be able to tell you what the medication is for and answer your questions. But you should learn what your pills look like and why you are taking them. This applies, of course, only if you are awake and alert.

Uncertainty about what nurses do and how the hospital system works can cause anxiety. Because the nursing profession has sometimes been distorted by the media, public perception of what nurses do frequently lags behind reality. In books and movies and on TV, nurses have been caricatured as bimbos or battle-axes, mere pillow fluffers, glorified maids, or physicians' "go-fers." Nothing could be further from the truth.

As students, nurses learn to look after patients in a variety of settings. They study physiology, anatomy, chemistry, pharmacology, psychology, and sociology. They use assessment skills developed through experience to watch for subtle changes in a patient's condition. They are responsible for administering potentially lethal drugs correctly. They are accountable for controlled drugs, including narcotics, which are kept locked up and are counted at the end of each shift. Nurses must notify doctors of significant patient problems. They act as patient advocates and share information with other personnel in the health care community, such as physical therapists and social workers.

WHO'S WHO IN THE NURSING HIERARCHY

About two-thirds of all nurses work in hospitals, where the average salary is $35,000. There are two basic categories of nurses:

▲ The Registered Nurse (RN)

▲ The Licensed Vocational Nurse (LVN) or Licensed Practical Nurse (LPN), depending on the state

REGISTERED NURSES

RNs complete either a four-year university program leading to a Bachelor of Science in Nursing (BSN) degree, a three-year diploma program, or a two-year associate degree. All must pass state board exams. RNs can specialize further by pursuing graduate degrees or specialized programs that lead to positions in advanced practice areas, such as nurse clinician, nurse practitioner, nurse midwife, or nurse anesthetist, or that prepare for teaching or administrative positions.

LICENSED VOCATIONAL NURSES

LVNs and LPNs most often complete a one- to two-year community college program. In clinical settings like hospitals, they do almost everything RNs do except take charge of a ward or perform certain procedures such as transfusing blood or injecting medications directly into intravenous lines. Some LVNs and LPNs return to school at a later date to become RNs.

NURSING ASSISTANTS

Certified Nursing Assistants (CNAs) help nurses in many hospitals. They take a short course—perhaps only two or three weeks—to learn the basics of lifting, turning, dressing, and bathing patients and how to take vital signs, including blood pressure. They are sometimes called "aides" or "techs," but do not do any technical procedures or give out medications. They are paid little more than minimum wage.

SPECIALTY NURSES

Nurse clinician or clinical nurse specialist (CNS)	*RNs with master's degrees in specialized areas such as maternal and child health, mental health, diabetes, and cardiac care in hospitals, clinics, and the community.*
Nurse practitioner (NP)	*RNs with an additional two years' post-degree training. NPs do almost everything doctors do. They take medical histories, diagnose and treat minor illnesses and injuries, and order and interpret lab tests and X-rays, referring clients to doctors if more intensive treatment is required.*
Nurse midwife (CNM, certified) nurse midwife	*CMNs provide prenatal care, supervise labor and normal deliveries, and provide post-partum care. They practice in hospitals, birth centers, and homes, and usually collaborate with obstetricians to whom they refer complicated cases.*
Nurse anesthetist	*Nurse anesthetists complete a program of at least two years in addition to their nursing degree and are then licensed to administer some types of anesthesia in certain situations or to assist an anesthesiologist.*

A CHANGING FIELD

It used to be easy to tell who the nurses were. They wore caps and white uniforms. Today their appearance varies greatly, depending on individual hospital policy. Some still require a standard uniform, but it most likely consists of a colored pantsuit. Caps have virtually disappeared. In many hospitals, nurses can wear any uniform of their choice, or even casual street clothes. Casual attire may be less threatening to patients, but can be frustrating and confusing as you struggle to find out who's who and to differentiate nurses from volunteers or lab technicians. While nurses must wear ID badges that show name and position, these have a way of becoming hidden behind a lapel.

Conventional appearances may not always prevail in hospitals in this era of individual rights and freedom of expression. Dress codes for nurses used to require short or pulled-back hair, minimal make-up, and no jewelry. Now nurses often wear long hair, polished nails, and dramatic jewelry, which can cause culture shock if you haven't been around hospitals lately. Aunt Sally from Sunrise, Iowa, may be in for a surprise if she is hospitalized while visiting Philadelphia and looked after by a nurse who has tattoos and dreadlocks.

An increasing number of nurses are male, and they may be straight or gay. It is not uncommon for a male nurse to be assigned to a female patient. If you object to this, you can request only female nurses. There is also an unwritten rule that a nurse never looks after anyone she/he knows personally, which poses a problem only in the smallest of hospitals serving a tiny population.

If you do not want a particular nurse assigned to you, speak to the charge nurse. He or she will accommodate your request if at all possible. On the other hand, a nurse may ask not to look after a certain patient. Nurses are human too and should not have to tolerate unacceptable behavior from patients, such as rudeness, intrusively personal questions, and, occasionally, inappropriate sexual behavior. Allowances are made for patients who are not fully able to control their actions due to dementia, disorientation, and various forms of mental illness. Nurses sometimes look after a difficult patient by taking turns. This prevents burnout.

Nursing is increasingly specialized today. A nurse who has spent years working in labor and delivery, for instance, would need to learn new skills and review his/her basic education if switched suddenly to a surgical or psychiatric floor. Nurses who work in emergency rooms, intensive care units, and recovery rooms occupy the most demanding positions. But no matter where she/he works, a nurse should be able to explain tests, procedures, and medications to you or find out if she/he doesn't know.

NURSING RESPONSIBILITIES

On most units, a nurse has six to eight patients, but in specialized units such as Intensive Care and Coronary Care, she/he may have only one or two. The pace is brisk on a hospital unit, and rare moments of calm can quickly change to frantic activity. As a patient, a technique you can use to get your needs met quickly is to consolidate your requests so they can be done in one fell swoop. For instance, if you need more pain medication but would also like more ice water, some tissues, and the room temperature adjusted, get all this done at the same time when the nurse is in the room.

AT THE START OF EACH SHIFT

A nurse begins the shift by checking on her/his patients and making sure that tubes, IV lines, and machines are working properly. The nurse or an aide takes vital signs—temperature, pulse, respirations, and blood pressure—for each patient. The nurse checks their charts for new doctors' orders such as changes in medication or new lab tests. The nurse either processes these her/himself or passes them to the charge nurse or unit clerk, depending on how the unit is organized. They then send messages by computer to the hospital pharmacy, labs, or central supply room.

COORDINATING CARE AND MEDICATIONS

You may need transportation to other parts of the hospital for tests, therapies or surgery. The nurse arranges this and fields phone calls from family members, doctors, and other hospital personnel. She/he checks your medication chart and portions out your medications for the shift. These are kept in locked cupboards outside your room or in a central location until needed. The nurse gives out extra medications, called "PRN medications," for pain, nausea, or other conditions as needed.

PAPERWORK

Patients being admitted or discharged require extra time and paperwork. When you are admitted, the nurse asks questions about your medical history and medications. Bring a list of your pills rather than the pills themselves. Your doctor may change your medication while you're in the hospital. Keep your answers brief and focused. Your nurse's time is limited, with endless details to attend to. Not least are the notes the nurse writes in each patient's chart every shift. Her/his only break may be twenty minutes to grab a sandwich.

STAFFING LEVELS

As a patient, you may notice a parade of different nurses looking after you. If you are in the hospital only two or three days, you may not get the same nurse twice. This is because many nurses choose to work part time in order to have more control over their schedules, juggle the demands of combining work with raising a family, or to minimize the stress of the job itself. A hospital may have its own pool of part-time or "relief" staff, or it may use nurses from various private agencies to fill gaps in staffing. This is not necessarily a negative thing in itself. Even nurses from outside agencies often work regularly in particular hospitals or units and become quite familiar with them. Charge nurses provide continuity and backup. Hospitals save money when they use part-time staff. Although they pay more for nurses from outside agencies, they do not, as a rule, pay any benefits to part-timers.

The severity of patients' conditions, plus staff cuts at many hospitals, means that workload stress for nurses has steadily increased in recent years. In this era of shrinking budgets and managed care, nurses are often considered the most expendable personnel in the hospital.

Poor staffing or an unexpectedly high patient "census" can result in a shift that consists of a mad dash from room to room doing the minimum, not by choice, but due to constraints of time and personnel. Patients able to afford it can hire private-duty nurses, aides, or "sitters" from agencies to ensure closer care, especially at night when staffing levels are lower.

UNLICENSED STAFF

A problematic area is the developing trend to use unlicensed personnel to perform tasks nurses traditionally do. These employees may be trained to carry out certain isolated procedures, such as checking blood sugars in diabetic patients, suctioning patients, or changing bandages, usually called "dressings." But they may lack the in-depth professional skills and judgment needed to assess the patients' needs.

A controversial ethical issue under scrutiny by nursing's professional associations is the need for hospitals to fully disclose to consumers the qualifications of the people caring for them. Most patients assume they will be looked after by fully qualified nurses. Says Claire Jordan, Executive Director of the Texas Nurses' Association, "There is a value conflict between nursing's emphasis on the whole patient and the economic, technically based and cost-saving agenda of managed care, where the emphasis is on doing the minimum." As a patient, you can always ask a caregiver what her or his title is and request that the RN or LVN assigned to you check on you frequently.

YOUR ROLE

What are your responsibilities as a patient or a concerned visitor? Ask questions. Take note of what is going on around you to the best of your ability. Be polite to the staff, help when you can, and, indeed, join the team. Learn the staff's names. Gifts of flowers, candy or fruit, or an appreciative card are appropriate if you feel you had good care. Be sure to read "Ten Tips for Patients" on page 55. Memorize them before you go to the hospital. They will help make your stay as tolerable as possible.

QUALITIES OF A GOOD NURSE

What makes a good nurse? A good nurse should:

▲ Possess basic professional qualities.

▲ Take time to explain things to you or find out if she/he doesn't know, or have the courtesy to tell you in advance if the doctor has ordered a new X-ray, made a change in medication, or even if you will be getting a new roommate.

▲ Be nonjudgmental about your lifestyle, even if it contributed to your current hospitalization. You may abuse drugs or alcohol, have a criminal record, or belong to a religion whose beliefs about medical treatment conflict with standard treatments, such as a religious prohibition on blood transfusions. It is not the nurse's role to judge you or discuss behavior with you unless you initiate such a discussion.

▲ Be a patient advocate and have your well-being uppermost in her/his mind.

▲ Pass on messages and phone calls you may have missed.

▲ Pace her/himself. A nurse cannot spend twenty minutes talking to one patient if this leaves her/him short of time and energy to check on other patients or talk to a patient who is upset and crying.

When we add the fact that nursing combines high responsibility with low control over working conditions, it is little wonder that hospital nursing is on record as one of the most demanding jobs possible. Yet most nurses care deeply about their patients and want them to get the best possible care. They often stay overtime or make a special effort to ensure that patients receive the attention they need.

Other Hospital Workers:

WHO DID YOU SAY YOU WERE?

Kim Collins was startled awake late at night by a man crouched at the foot of her bed. It was Kim's second night following knee surgery. "What are you doing?" she called. "It's all right, Ma'am," he replied. "Maintenance sent me. I'm just fixing the control on this bed." Kim had been unable to raise the head of the bed by using the control button on the bedrail that connected to rods under the bed. Though the repair was overdue, the timing was inappropriate. Worse, no one had told her that maintenance would be coming.

Exposure to an almost constant parade of personnel is routine for most hospital patients. It can be a challenge to learn who's who, to differentiate between a volunteer in a white coat and a lab technician in a pink one. A respiratory technician may be required to wear a dark blue pantsuit but a nurse may buy a similar uniform. Ideally, all hospital employees should wear highly visible ID badges, but in reality these are often hard to read and may be hidden behind folds of clothing or under stethoscopes.

CLERKS

Among the first personnel you may encounter are clerical staff, who range from the admitting clerk who is your initial contact with the hospital, to the unit clerk whose function is described in Chapter Four.

LABORATORY TECHNICIANS

Lab technicians are trained to take blood samples for tests. Some hospitals also have an "IV team" who circulate throughout the hospital to start intravenous lines and draw blood. Other lab technicians work in the hospital laboratories, which are usually divided into hematology, chemistry, microbiology, the blood bank, and other specialty areas.

IMAGING TECHNICIANS

The radiology, or X-ray, department has a staff of technicians, some of whom are certified to operate sophisticated equipment. They are called imaging technicians and take courses that last several months or more to learn how to operate ultrasound machines, computerized axial tomography (CAT) scanners, and magnetic resonance imaging (MRI) scanners. These provide three-dimensional views of body parts that yield detailed information to greatly improve diagnosis. Nuclear medicine technicians assist specialists (MDs) in nuclear medicine with scans involving radioactive substances placed in the body to detect cancer or help to cure it. Radiologists, who are MDs, are ultimately responsible for interpreting X-ray pictures and information.

EKG TECHNICIANS

EKG technicians do electrocardiograms. They also help with various stress tests that yield valuable information on how the heart is functioning. These include treadmill tests, the use of Holter monitors (worn by patients for a period of days while going about their daily activities), and echocardiograms that measure blood flow through major blood vessels.

PHARMACY STAFF

The pharmacy is staffed by pharmacists, who complete a five-year university program, and pharmacy technicians, who replace supplies, take stock, and deliver medications to the units or floors. The list of drugs a hospital carries is called its "formulary" and may differ somewhat from hospital to hospital.

HEALTH EDUCATORS

In many hospitals, health educators provide specialized teaching. Not all are nurses; dietitians could provide nutritional information. Physical therapists might coordinate exercise programs for post–heart-attack patients. Nurse clinicians are often involved in education. One example would be in the area of diabetic teaching, where the nurse would develop educational materials and programs for patients newly diagnosed with diabetes. An educator might use tapes, videos, and books and also serve as a resource person whom you may contact at any time for help.

INFECTION CONTROL

Most hospitals have a nurse or other professional who tracks any infections that occur in patients after they are hospitalized. These are called "nosocomial" infections. Infection control also develops and monitors prevention and control strategies.

REHABILITATION SPECIALISTS

Rehabilitation is the area of medicine that deals with patients who need long-term care. They may have had strokes, traumatic accidents, or severe head injuries that seriously impair their ability to speak, think, and function normally. Many professionals are involved in the care of these patients:

- ▲ Physical therapists (PTs) work with a broad spectrum of patients, from those who are severely incapacitated to those who may need only some coaching in how to walk with crutches.

- ▲ Respiratory therapists (RTs) use various types of oxygen masks, inhalers, and other equipment to help patients who have breathing difficulties.

- ▲ Speech therapists assess a patient's ability to talk, swallow, and eat.

- ▲ Occupational therapists (OTs) train patients in activities of daily living, such as dressing themselves and cooking.

- ▲ Recreational therapists provide diversionary as well as educational activities.

- ▲ Orthopedic techs, or orthotic specialists, design and make devices such as artificial limbs and braces.

SOCIAL WORKERS

Many hospitals employ social workers, sometimes called case managers, who interact among patients, families, insurers, and other agencies, particularly when there are special needs involved. They can:

- ▲ Arrange for placement in a rehabilitation facility, such as for a patient who is too stable to remain in an acute care hospital but is not yet ready to go home.

- ▲ Arrange nursing home placement and home care visits for those who need ongoing support after they leave the hospital.

- ▲ Handle many other problems, from referrals to other helping agencies, to finding housing for financially strapped families from out of town.

PASTORAL CARE STAFF

Hospital chaplains, or pastoral care professionals, address the spiritual and emotional needs of patients and their loved ones. The availability of this service varies with the size and type of hospital, but all hospitals have a list of on-call people who can serve as friendly visitors, provide solace in time of death, or discuss your concerns. Religious denomination, or lack thereof, is of secondary importance—these services are available to all patients.

MENTAL HEALTH STAFF

Many hospitals employ mental health professionals to help assess and assist patients in certain circumstances. Psychologists can help a patient who appears to be deeply depressed. They can design learning programs for brain-damaged or cognitively impaired patients. Licensed counselors can help establish and facilitate support groups for patients and families that often provide ongoing help after a patient leaves the hospital. Such groups include survivors of strokes, cancer patients, and those with substance abuse problems and chronic illness. Medical social workers can assist newly discharged psychiatric patients with housing and community support organizations.

PATIENT REPRESENTATIVES

The hospital often employs a patient representative, sometimes called a patient advocate or "ombudsman" (from a Scandinavian term for "mediator"). Some may have backgrounds in social work or pastoral care. Their mandate varies widely from hospital to hospital. In some cases, patient representatives may be impartial observers who can argue for the patient's best interests. But in other cases, the patient representative is little more than a public relations employee who upholds the hospital's status quo. All may have divided loyalties, given the conflict of interest between helping you and protecting the institution. A good patient advocacy system provides quick access to the hospital administrator and various hospital committees. You may find an informal advocate in a friend, family member, social worker, nurse, doctor, or lawyer, who can make representations on your behalf when there is a problem or grievance. Often such problems arise from lack of clear information and the resulting misunderstanding. Problems that occur can often be settled by arbitration rather than legal action. In some situations, a patient may be asked to voluntarily sign a form to agree to arbitration rather than resorting to a lawsuit.

OTHER HOSPITAL STAFF

Behind-the-scenes departments like public relations, accounting, finance, research and development, fund-raising, payroll, benefits, and employee health contain personnel you probably never see. As a patient, you may be more aware of housekeeping, security, and food services staff. The latter department includes the employees who prepare and deliver meals, the dietitians who plan them, and the nutritionists who design diets for unique health needs.

Hospitals used to have porters, or "runners," who carried specimens to the lab, delivered needed equipment to the unit, transported patients by wheelchair or gurney, and ran many other errands. Today they are a vanishing breed, as most departments, from X-ray to the lab, use their own personnel to fill this role.

Last but not least are the volunteers who, while often invisible, save the hospital many hours of labor and expense. They answer phones, escort patients, deliver flowers, give directions, and are always appreciated by the busy hospital staff.

What should you do if you don't know who's who? Simply ask what department they are from and what they have come to do. It's part of their job to identify themselves and it's certainly your right to know. In rare instances, impostors have impersonated employees. If you have any doubts, ask for the charge nurse who can quietly check to verify a suspicious person's ID.

There is no doubt that it is stressful for you as a patient to deal constantly with a stream of unfamiliar faces when coping with hospitalization and illness. Each has a vital role to play in your care, however. But if you are disturbed by too many surprise visits from housekeeping staff at strange hours or technicians who barge in unannounced, you can ask that a sign be placed on your door requesting all visitors, staff or not, to knock and/or check at the nurses' station first before entering your room. This can help postpone less crucial interruptions to a more convenient time. After all, hospitals ideally should be restful places.

Patients:

SPECIAL ISSUES TO CONSIDER

Patients often have special concerns when hospitalized. Added to the stress of the illness is the disruption in your usual lifestyle. You want to do all you can to ensure appropriate care, maintain contact with supportive family and friends, continue habits and practices that are important to you, and keep in touch with your usual activities.

ADVANCE DIRECTIVE

An advance directive is either a living will or a durable health care power of attorney, or both. A living will informs others what medical treatment you desire or do not desire if you become permanently unconscious or terminally ill and are unable to communicate decisions. If unsure about a living will, discuss its implications with your doctor, attorney, or a pastoral care professional ahead of time. Although we may like to think we can fix everything, there are many times when extreme measures such as cardiopulmonary resuscitation (CPR) may not be appropriate. For example, in the case of an eighty-five-year-old terminally ill patient with cancer who has a cardiac arrest, it may be an undignified and traumatic procedure. In many cases, especially in the elderly, CPR is unsuccessful or results only in broken ribs and a reduction of oxygen to the brain, causing further damage. If a "Do Not Resuscitate" (DNR) order is desired, it must be a written doctor's order on your chart. It must be renewed after a set period of time and every time you are transferred to a new floor or are readmitted. A durable health care power of attorney lets you appoint someone to make decisions about your health care should you become incapable

WHAT TO CONSIDER
WHEN CHOOSING SOMEONE TO MAKE
HEALTH CARE DECISIONS FOR YOU

▲ *The person to whom you give power of attorney for health care decisions must be over eighteen years of age.*

▲ *He or she must not be one of your health care providers, such as a doctor, home health agency employee, residential care employee, etc.*

▲ *The individual must be willing to take on responsibility for making health care decisions. You must inform them and give them the same signed copy of the health care power of attorney that you give your doctor.*

▲ *The individual you name should know what is contained in your living will (technically, a directive to physicians), particularly in regard to the use of heroic measures to prolong life.*

▲ *Your connection with the person to whom you give power of attorney for health care decisions should be one of long-term commitment, not someone with whom you have a relatively short-term, uncommitted relationship. Examples are a spouse, sibling, good friend, adult child, or long-term partner. If a marriage is dissolved, the formerly designated spouse no longer has health care power of attorney.*

▲ *You can revoke your choice orally or in writing at any time and appoint a new individual.*

These forms are not required or mandatory, but are becoming a routine part of the admission process. They can be changed at any time. If you have these documents already, you should give copies to the hospital each time you are admitted.

VISITING POLICIES

Visiting policies are sometimes an issue. When you are in a private room, most hospitals now allow unlimited visiting and a significant other can stay overnight on a folding bed or cot. More liberal visiting policies for children are now in effect, within reason. It is not a good idea to expose an infant or very young child to the hospital environment unnecessarily. Nor should toddlers crawl on the floor or touch equipment. Far from the pristine environments you may imagine them to be, hospitals are far more germ-filled than the average home.

HOLISTIC THERAPIES

You may have an interest in holistic or alternative health beliefs and practices, as opposed to standard Western medical practices that are sometimes referred to as "biomedicine." Much is still unknown about the mind–body connection and its role in healing. Alternative health is gaining in interest and acceptance in our society as health consumers become more involved in their own care. This awareness of other ways of healing has percolated through American life since the 1960s. It has picked up momentum in recent years as consumers have become uneasy about escalating health care costs and sweeping changes, such as managed care, and more skeptical about traditional health care. A holistic approach takes the whole person into consideration. Your emotions, significant relationships, material and financial situation, worries, fears, and concerns, as well as physical symptoms, are all important factors in the healing process.

Many alternative heath approaches can be used within the hospital. Certainly meditation and visualization techniques are easy to apply while lying in a hospital bed. One woman spent several hours in labor focusing on favorite pieces of music as a form of self-hypnosis. Any mandalas, crystals, pictures, or tapes that can help you cope and feel calm are beneficial. After all, more traditional religious items, such as rosaries, have always been accepted.

Physical applications, such as massage, also have their place in the hospital, as long as they do not impact negatively on surgical incisions, injured areas, or equipment such as IVs and traction. Yoga exercises, such as breathing, can be helpful. Pranic healing requires no contact with the patient. The practitioner works on the energy body or field and uses "prana," the life force available from the sun, air, and earth to heal physical and emotional imbalances. As you heal the bioplasmic mind–body, you also heal the body. Pranic healing sets out to remove the disease energies and reenergize with the life force or prana. Acupuncture and traditional Chinese medicine have gained wider acceptance. Western medicine views the body as a machine. When something goes wrong, the solution is to fix, replace, or remove the broken part. Eastern medicine sees the body as a whole entity and focuses more on prevention and harmony.

If you use herbal teas, vitamins, and other natural food products at home, check with your doctor so that continued use of these in hospital does not interfere with the treatment plan. In many cases, you may continue to use them. Most hospitals can now provide vegetarian meals without blinking an eye.

Journal writing can be therapeutic as an outlet for your feelings, thoughts, and anxieties. Headphones tuned to favorite music, from opera to country, can be soothing and distracting. Prayer and meditation are beneficial. A number of studies show that patients prayed for by others often have a smoother course of recovery. Some practices, such as chanting or burning candles or incense, may be unacceptable as they may disturb roommates or patients in adjacent rooms, not to mention that they may violate the hospital fire and safety codes.

Some doctors and nurses may be somewhat unsupportive, dismissive, or even faintly scornful of alternative health practices in some situations. But for some patients, these practices provide hope and emotional sustenance. People who have chronic illnesses often use alternative therapies, not necessarily to cure the disease but to live with it more easily.

WHAT MAKES A GOOD PATIENT?

Your health care team will consider you a good patient if you display these qualities:

- ▲ Are polite and use "please" and "thank you" when possible.
- ▲ Make needs known as they develop. "You didn't bring me my pain medication!" one patient said accusingly as a new nurse walked into the room. "But you didn't ask for

any," the nurse replied, as he went to get it. The nurse understood that the patient was anxious and fatigued. When he returned with the medication, he gently reminded the patient to ask for pain relief whenever he felt he needed it and to not wait until he was in great discomfort or until a staff member asked him if he needed it.

▲ Are somewhat adaptable. If you need to be moved to another room because a roommate has developed an infection that requires isolation, you accept this as being in your own best interest.

▲ Have read up on your medical condition and can ask informed questions.

▲ Understand that others may also have needs. For instance, someone down the hall needs pain medication, which takes precedence over your need for an extra straw.

▲ Try to comply with the therapies offered. If it's time to go to X-ray, stop your phone conversation. If the physical therapy scheduled daily is met with "No, I don't feel like it right now," you not only throw the therapist's schedule out of whack, but also deprive yourself of its benefit.

The hospital staff appreciates a good patient. As in other areas of life, a little common sense and give and take go a long way to smooth a hospital stay.

WHAT MAKES A GOOD SUPPORTER?

A friend or relative can provide moral support in these ways:

▲ Just by silently being there.

▲ By finding out information for you.

▲ By doing things you cannot do for yourself, such as providing reading material, looking up a phone number, or bringing in extra toiletries or clothes from home.

▲ By reminding you of questions to ask.

▲ By not trying to do too much.

A support person can become a negative factor if she/he pesters the staff, gets in the way physically or emotionally, brings in food or drink you are not supposed to have, or demands special treatment for you. A young woman was upset when her beloved grandmother was hospitalized with a stroke. She was helpful to her, but badgered the staff constantly. At the beginning of one shift, she even went so far as to say to the nurse looking after her grandmother, "You'll answer her light first." The nurse had to state firmly that she had seven other patients to look after and had to treat them equally, without favoritism. The nurse was resentful of the visitor telling her what her priorities should be and how to do her job.

Overbearing and demanding visitors can cause friction with the staff. This can actually impact negatively on the patient's care if staff avoid entering that patient's room due to the unpleasant behavior of those visitors. A little give and take between visitors and staff can work wonders and results in all concerned working in harmony for the patient's well-being.

TEN TIPS FOR PATIENTS

A hospital stay is seldom enjoyable. To ensure that you get the best possible treatment, remember the following:

1. *Know what treatment your doctor plans, including all possible outcomes, side effects, and length of stay.*

2. *Have as much testing as possible done ahead of time as an outpatient. This reduces in-hospital time and costs. Check into the hospital in the afternoon and leave before noon to avoid being charged for an extra day.*

3. *Leave valuables at home. Theft can occur in the hospital. Your health insurance cards, basic toiletries, and a few dollars should be all you need. Do not bring credit cards, jewelry, or large amounts of cash.*

4. *Bring a list of your medications, but leave your pills at home. Your doctor may make changes in your medication for the duration of your hospital stay.*

(continued)

5. *Be polite to the staff. They are not your personal servants and most work hard.*

6. *Be considerate of your roommate by keeping TV and radio noise to a minimum and limiting visitors to one at a time.*

7. *Don't be surprised if you have a different nurse every day. Shifts change every eight to twelve hours, many nurses work part-time, and hospitals often employ nurses from agencies. Each nurse usually looks after several patients.*

8. *Be aware that each shift is supervised by a "charge nurse" who is responsible for everything that happens during the shift. If you have questions your nurse can't answer, ask to speak to the charge nurse.*

9. *You may have nonmedical questions related to your insurance, lack thereof, post-hospital treatment, or emotional well-being. Ask to speak to the social services department, a patient representative, patient advocate, or chaplain.*

10. *If you have major concerns or complaints, contact the hospital administrator. It is part of his or her job to address them*

Take responsibility for your hospital stay. Become informed. Keep asking questions. It's your body, your life, and your rights.

Payment:
NO FREE LUNCH

Lynn grew up in England where, as in most of the developed world, the government provides good health care almost free of direct charge to the patient, although it is paid for through taxes. She married an American and moved to the United States, where her reaction to the health system was one of "culture shock."

"I don't understand why health insurance has to be so complicated here," she complained to her friend Barbara.

"Never mind," said Barbara, "Most Americans don't understand it either."

More than likely, you are covered by some form of health insurance that pays for some—if not all—of the hospital bill. There are hundreds of different plans and what they offer varies tremendously. The great majority of patients have health coverage through their employers, although some individuals have their own plans and pay the entire cost of their premiums. Medicare is a federally administered plan that covers those over age sixty-five as well as some Americans with disabilities of a chronic nature, such as kidney failure requiring dialysis. Medicaid is a program for those living below the poverty line that each state administers, setting its own criteria for coverage.

"SCHOLARSHIP" PATIENTS

Some Americans fall through the cracks when it comes to health insurance. You may be working, but not covered through your employer and unable to pay for coverage due to low earnings. Yet you earn too much to qualify for Medicaid. Many hospitals accept a limited number of uninsured patients as "scholarship" or "charity" cases. A number of factors influence a hospital's ability to accept uninsured patients. Those who are young and likely to return to a productive life, and those who have a place to go after discharge are most likely to get free care. Each hospital has its own criteria for making these decisions, based on its funding and resources. The doctors likely to treat these patients must also agree to give pro bono services.

The ultimate decision rests with the financial end of the hospital admissions department. A number of charitable funds exist to help in these situations, but their availability varies greatly from one community to another. Specialized case managers called "community liaison" nurses often help coordinate ongoing care. For instance, if you are past the acute stage of an illness but still require further rehabilitation, a nurse liaison can search out a facility willing to accept you.

HOSPITAL BILLING PRACTICES

Most hospitals are involved in a number of different billing arrangements. Sometimes the hospital bills the insurer directly, or it may bill you. In either case, you should receive a fully itemized bill for verification. If you are in a managed care plan, such as an HMO, or are covered by Medicare, you may get only a statement of what your care cost. A hospital "accepts assignment" for Medicare. This means it agrees to be paid by the Health Care Financing Administration (HCFA), which administers Medicare. Many Medicare recipients are also covered by supplemental insurance, since Medicare seldom covers the entire cost of treatment. If you send a bill to your insurer for payment, in addition to a copy of the bill include photocopies of your policy's title page, both sides of your insurance card, and a properly filled out claim form.

Medicaid is a program administered by each state to provide care for those under sixty-five who have very low incomes. As eligibility varies greatly from state to state, contact your state Medicaid office for information.

Some insurance plans require that the patient pay the bill and then submit claim forms for reimbursement.

Hospital billing cycles vary, but you will probably get a bill within a couple of weeks of discharge. Go over it with a fine-tooth comb, preferably with someone who understands medical terminology. There are a number of things to watch for when examining a hospital bill. Common billing errors include the following:

▲ Medications never prescribed for your condition

▲ Anesthesia charges for women who had unmedicated childbirth

▲ Duplicate charges

Sometimes hospitals itemize too much. This practice, called "unbundling" or "debulking," involves breaking down routine procedures into separate parts so that the sum of the individual charges is greater than the whole. Ask for an explanation of any puzzling items or "miscellaneous" charges. Companies that help people check the accuracy of their hospital bills are called "cost review" or "medical review" services.

REDUCING HOSPITAL COSTS

Here are some tips on how to reduce costs:

▲ Get a copy of the hospital's "usual and customary charges," "published charges," or "established charges," which include such basic items as room rates.

▲ Preauthorize your hospitalization with your insurer, a requirement in most cases now.

▲ Prebank blood for yourself or have family and friends do so. This can eliminate the higher charges for drawing blood and checking it for blood type once you have been admitted to the hospital.

▲ Have any required tests done as an outpatient before a planned admission.

▲ Question any doctor's fees for admission and discharge. Usually these are unnecessary fees since no work is involved.

▲ Arrive after noon and leave before noon to avoid being charged for an extra day.

▲ Do not accept charges for any tests that had to be repeated due to someone's error.

If an insurer turns down your claim, get your doctor to contact them and verify the claim or ask to speak to the insurance company's doctor.

If you are uninsured or only partially insured, it is possible to arrange to put down a deposit and then pay the remaining bill in installments. You do not have to pay the entire bill prior to being discharged. Payment schedules can be worked out with the patient accounts office.

If you have questions about your bill, contact the patient accounts office. You can also talk to the administrator or a representative. The administration and patient representatives are there to address your problems and make sure that you are treated fairly. If you do not receive satisfaction, call your state insurance regulator's office with your questions.

PART II
Understanding
Technical Matters

CHAPTER 8: BASIC BODY SYSTEMS: A Short Review 63
The Cardiovascular System 63
The Respiratory System 65
The Digestive System 66
The Renal System 67
The Musculoskeletal System..67
The Neurological System..68
The Metabolic System...69
The Immune System 71

**CHAPTER 9: MEDICAL EQUIPMENT AND
PROCEDURES: A User-Friendly Guide 72**
The Cardiovascular System 74
The Respiratory System 84
The Digestive System 88
The Renal System 91
The Musculoskeletal System..94
The Neurological System..97
The Metabolic System...97
Pain Control 98

**CHAPTER 10: DRUGS: What You Don't Know
Can Hurt You 100**
Generic and Brand Names 100
Prescribing Drugs at the Hospital 100
The Formulary 101
Delivering and Administering Medications 101
Tips for Appropriate Use 102
The Cardiovascular System 102
The Respiratory System 105
The Digestive System 106
The Renal System 106
The Musculoskeletal System..107
The Neurological System..107
The Metabolic System...110
The Immune System 111
Drugs Frequently Prescribed in the Hospital 112
Using Drugs Wisely..113

8

Basic Body Systems:
A SHORT REVIEW

It is all too true that most of us know more about our car engines and computers than about how our bodies function. Whether through lack of interest, fear, denial, or a lingering Puritanism, most of us put off learning about how the interrelated systems that make up our bodies work—until something goes wrong. We then scramble for information, often under the pressure of panic and time constraints.

This section is a basic review of body systems organized under a number of headings, although this approach is a little like attempting to see Disneyland in ten minutes. The systems covered include the following:

i) Cardiovascular

ii) Respiratory

iii) Digestive

iv) Renal

v) Musculoskeletal

vi) Nervous

vii) Metabolic

viii) Immune System

THE CARDIOVASCULAR SYSTEM

The cardiovascular system, made up of the heart and blood vessels, pumps blood to all the cells of the body. Blood contains the oxygen that is necessary to sustain human life.

THE HEART

The heart is a hollow, muscular structure divided into two halves, each with two chambers. The two upper chambers are the atria and the two lower are the ventricles. Valves control the blood's passage between the chambers. The right side of the heart receives blood from the body through the veins and pumps it into the lungs. In the lungs, carbon dioxide is removed from the blood, and the blood receives a fresh supply of oxygen. The oxygenated blood returns from the lungs to the left side of the heart and is pumped to all the tissues of the body via the arteries (tissues cannot live without oxygen). The blood supply to the heart itself is provided by the right and left coronary arteries.

Chemicals in the heart's cells create electrical charges that control the heart's activity. The main "pacemaker" is the sinus node, located in the right atrium. From there, an electrical impulse passes to a "relay station" located at the junction of the right atrium and ventricle, called the A-V node. And from the A-V node, it passes on through specialized bundles of cells running along the wall separating the two ventricles. These electrical impulses are what an electrocardiogram picks up. It prints a graph of heart activity that provides valuable diagnostic information.

BLOOD

Blood is made up of cells and a fluid called plasma. Red blood cells carry oxygen and are manufactured in the bone marrow. Hemoglobin is the red pigment of the blood and is composed of protein and iron. It picks up oxygen in the lungs and transports it to the rest of the body. White blood cells fight infection and injury. Platelets are blood cells that stick together to promote healing when a wound occurs.

COMMON CARDIOVASCULAR PROBLEMS

Many conditions can affect the cardiovascular system. The most common problem is atherosclerosis, caused by fatty deposits in the arteries. The arteries become blocked and narrowed, reducing blood supply. When blood supply to the heart is greatly inadequate, the result is often chest pain (angina). A heart attack is called a "myocardial infarction" (MI). It refers to a blockage in a major artery that supplies the heart muscle (myocardium).

Other heart problems are caused by valves that thicken, wear out, or become scarred from infection. Electrical conduction disturbances due to chemical imbalances in the heart can cause faulty heart rhythm (arrhythmia), leading to reduced blood supply and oxygen. Congestive heart failure occurs when the heart is no longer able to pump an adequate supply of blood to meet the demands of the body. A stroke occurs when there is a sudden interference with the circulation of blood in the brain, usually caused by bleeding or blockage of an artery. Diseases of the blood vessels include inflammation, which can cause blood clots to form.

THE RESPIRATORY SYSTEM

The respiratory system includes the mouth, nose, pharynx, and trachea, which forks into two bronchi (tubes), connecting to the two lungs.

THE LUNGS

Inside the lungs, the bronchi branch into many smaller bronchioles. Like clusters of grapes, some 300 million alveoli, or tiny sacs, cling to the bronchioles. They exchange oxygen and carbon dioxide in the blood. Fine hairs called "cilia" line the entire respiratory tract. The lungs are elastic and expand and contract with the help of the muscles of the diaphragm.

COMMON RESPIRATORY PROBLEMS

Many illnesses can affect the respiratory tract. The common cold is caused by viruses that infect the mucous membranes of the mouth and nose. Bronchitis can be viral or bacterial and acute or chronic. Cigarette smoke and air pollutants are common bronchial irritants. Pneumonia is inflammation of the lung by viral or bacterial invasion. This causes fluids to move into the alveoli, which become waterlogged. In emphysema, the alveoli become thickened and inelastic so that they must expand to their maximum to function at all and cannot expand further. This makes them ineffective in the exchange of oxygen and carbon dioxide. Asthma is caused by muscle spasm in the bronchi resulting from an allergic response to something in the environment. It causes difficult breathing.

THE DIGESTIVE SYSTEM

Food passes from the stomach, where hydrochloric acid begins the digestion process, to the small intestine, where it is completed. In the process, proteins are broken down into amino acids, fats into fatty acids, and glycerol and carbohydrates into glucose. Digestion is controlled by hormones. After digestion, waste products pass through the colon (large intestine) and are eliminated through the rectum.

LIVER

The liver is the body's main processing factory. It stores glucose, the body's main energy supplier, makes vitamins and blood clotting agents, creates bile, and reuses old blood cells that have been broken down in the spleen. The liver also detoxifies harmful substances.

GALLBLADDER

The gallbladder stores bile, which breaks down food in the intestine and helps excrete liver wastes.

PANCREAS

The pancreas produces pancreatic juice that neutralizes stomach acids and contains many digestive enzymes. It also produces insulin, which regulates the amount of sugar in the body.

COMMON GASTROINTESTINAL PROBLEMS

Common digestive problems include stomach ulcers, caused by bacteria wearing away the protective lining of the stomach, and appendicitis, inflammation of a tiny, worm-like projection of the large intestine. The gallbladder may become inflamed and gallstones may form. The colon, or large intestine, through which waste products pass, may develop growths called polyps, among other problems.

THE RENAL SYSTEM

KIDNEYS

The kidneys regulate the amount of water, salt, and acids in the body. Each kidney is composed of close to a million tiny nephrons (filters), fed by blood from the renal artery. Large blood cells, platelets, and proteins are stopped by the filter and returned to the body's circulation through the renal vein. The remaining liquid is broken down and filtered out by the kidneys. The waste product, urine, is carried by two ureters to the bladder and from there to the urethra, where it passes from the body.

COMMON RENAL SYSTEM PROBLEMS

The renal system can fall prey to a number of disorders, including infection, inadequate blood supply, inflammation, obstruction, and total failure. Renal failure may be acute, which is usually reversible if treated promptly, or chronic, treated by dialysis or transplant.

THE MUSCULOSKELETAL SYSTEM

BONES

There are 206 bones in the normal adult body. Bone is one of the most biologically active tissues and is made of collagen, a tough protein upon which calcium and mineral salts are deposited.

MUSCLES, TENDONS, AND LIGAMENTS

Muscles and bones are held together by tendons. There are three different types of muscle:

▲ Skeletal (voluntary)

▲ Smooth (involuntary)

▲ Cardiac (made up of linked fibers that contract in unison)

JOINTS

Joints are where bones meet. They are held together by ligaments and oiled by synovial fluid to reduce friction. The bearing surfaces of joints also have a lining of cartilage.

COMMON MUSCULOSKELETAL PROBLEMS

Common musculoskeletal problems include degeneration of joints caused by arthritis. Osteoarthritis causes wear and tear through a loss of the smooth tissue covering the joint surfaces and the forming of rough bone deposits. Rheumatoid arthritis is an inflammation of the connective tissue of the joints. These diseases account for many of the hip and knee replacements, in which damaged joints are replaced by synthetic ones, that are performed each year. Osteoporosis, a thinning of the bones; gout, a painful buildup of chemical crystal deposits around a joint; and muscle tears and strains, as well as bone fractures and dislocations are some of the most frequently experienced musculoskeletal conditions.

THE NEUROLOGICAL SYSTEM

The neurological system is composed of the brain, spinal cord, and nerves.

NERVES

Cerebrospinal fluid bathes the brain and spinal cord. Thirty-one pairs of nerves spring from the spinal cord, each leading to a specific part of the body. Motor pathways carry stimuli from the brain to the organs down through the spinal cord. Sensory pathways from the skin and other organs go up to the brain through the spinal cord.

Nerve cells (neurons) process information from outside and regulate this incoming information. There are 10 billion neurons in the body. The transmitting part is the nerve fiber (axon), while the receiving part is called the dendrite. Layers of fat called myelin sheaths are wrapped around the nerve fibers to protect them. Breakdown in the biochemical processes involved in myelin formation can lead to such diseases as multiple sclerosis.

NERVE IMPULSES

Nerve impulses are electrical waves. The electrical activity in a neuron is determined by electrically charged ions of potassium and sodium in the fluid in and around the cells. Chemical transmitters cross the gap (synapse), where two neurons meet. Examples of these transmitters are acetylcholine, norepinephrine, serotonin, and dopamine. Balance is all-important. In the case of dopamine, for instance, too little contributes to Parkinson's disease, while too much is believed to be a factor in schizophrenia.

PERIPHERAL NERVOUS SYSTEM

The peripheral nervous system, consisting of other nerves found throughout the body, is made up of the sympathetic and parasympathetic systems. They balance each other. The sympathetic nervous system stimulates the body, as in the "fight or flight" reflex, making it extra alert. It speeds up the heart rate, dilates the bronchi, and tenses the muscles. The parasympathetic system relaxes the muscles and bronchi and slows down the heart rate.

BRAIN

The cerebral cortex, or outer covering of the brain, interprets sensory information and is divided into two hemispheres and several lobes. The cerebellum controls motor skills and balance. The thalamus relays sensory information to the cortex and helps concentration. The hypothalamus controls desires such as hunger and sex and regulates the body's heat-sensing mechanism and the emotions. It also controls the endocrine system, a series of hormone-secreting glands throughout the body.

Major diseases of the nervous system include epilepsy, multiple sclerosis, Parkinson's disease, meningitis, and encephalitis, as well as spinal cord trauma.

THE METABOLIC SYSTEM

The metabolic system regulates many body functions through the actions of hormones that affect a number of glands and organs. When these hormones are in a state of imbalance, problems can occur.

An endocrine, or ductless, gland releases its hormones directly into the bloodstream. Exocrine glands secrete their hormones via ducts and have a more local effect. Examples of the latter are the digestive juices and sweat glands. The pituitary, thyroid, parathyroid, and adrenal glands are all endocrine, while the pancreas is both endocrine and exocrine.

PITUITARY GLAND

The hypothalamus receives conscious and unconscious impulses and sends out signals through nerves and hormones that travel in the bloodstream. As the master gland, the hypothalamus controls the pituitary gland. Among the hormones produced by the pituitary gland are human growth hormone, the sex hormones, and the hormones that stimulate the thyroid and adrenal glands. There are feedback mechanisms between the pituitary and most of the other glands. The pituitary gland releases hormones that stimulate these glands. When the glands have enough, they send signals back to the pituitary to stop. The pituitary's message to one of its target glands causes that gland in turn to send a message to specific organs or tissues.

THYROID GLAND

Thyroxine in the thyroid gland speeds up or slows down the body's metabolism, the rate at which the body burns energy and transforms food into body components. Problems can occur if it's out of sync. The parathyroid gland, embedded in the thyroid, regulates calcium, which is important for the function of muscles, nerves, and bones.

ADRENAL GLANDS

The adrenal glands above the kidneys produce corticosteroids that help the anti-inflammatory response in the body.

PANCREAS

The pancreas produces insulin to control sugar levels. Diabetes results when the pancreas fails to produce enough insulin, although it is also a digestive organ.

COMMON METABOLIC PROBLEMS

Common problems of the metabolic system include thyroid disease and tumors.

THE IMMUNE SYSTEM

The immune system protects the body against disease. Although the skin and mucous membranes are the first line of defense, the spleen, bone marrow, lymph nodes, and lymphatic cells form this system that protects you against harmful foreign substances such as bacteria and viruses. The white blood cells that fight these invaders develop from stem cells in the bone marrow. The thymus gland is the control organ of the immune system, directing the formation of white cells that gather in the lymph nodes and spleen, which enlarge if infection is present. At infection sites, an inflammatory response occurs, triggered by these white cells, which causes redness, swelling, and heat as they fight infection.

IMMUNE SYSTEM DISORDERS

There are a number of autoimmune diseases in which the body's immune system attacks healthy cells. Among the most common are rheumatoid arthritis and lupus. Rheumatoid arthritis is a chronic disease of the body's connective tissue where an allergic reaction to some component of the patient's own tissues causes swelling, stiffness, and pain in the joints. Lupus is a disease of the connective tissues and collagen that can manifest itself in fever, weakness, skin rashes, sensitivity to sunlight, and, in severe cases, damage to the kidneys and nervous system.

In acquired immune deficiency syndrome (AIDS), the human immunodeficiency virus (HIV) attacks the immune system. As a virus, it directs the host cell it invades to ignore normal functioning and give all its attention to reproducing the virus itself. Those who carry the virus may be symptom-free for years and then manifest flu-like symptoms, fever, diarrhea, and fatigue. When death occurs, it is most often due to other infections, such as pneumonia, that take advantage of the body's defective immune system.

Medical Equipment and Procedures:
A USER-FRIENDLY GUIDE

Tubes, wires, flashing monitors, ringing alarms—no wonder hospitals are intimidating. But there is a rationale for every item used. What follows is a list of equipment explained in non-technical terms. It is by no means a comprehensive list of items, but discusses those most commonly used.

This section is organized under headings based on the main body systems. However, these systems are deeply interconnected, as is the equipment. Many of the same items are used in the treatment of different illnesses. For example, a patient with a ruptured appendix may have an intravenous line, a drainage tube, and a Foley catheter. Another patient with a fractured leg and pneumonia may also have an IV, traction equipment, and oxygen delivered through nasal cannula.

In addition to the headings that correspond to the body systems, such as the cardiovascular and neurological systems, there is an additional heading that lists equipment used in pain control.

THE CARDIOVASCULAR SYSTEM
▲ Blood Pressure Cuff and Stethoscope
▲ Blood Transfusions
▲ Central Lines
▲ Crash Cart
▲ Defibrillators
▲ Electrocardiogram (EKG or ECG)
▲ Implanted Catheters
▲ Intravenous (IV) Lines
▲ IV Pumps

THE CARDIOVASCULAR SYSTEM (CONT'D)

▲ Needles and Syringes

▲ Saline Locks

▲ Secondary IV Lines

▲ Telemetry

THE RESPIRATORY SYSTEM

▲ Airway Tubes

▲ Chest Tubes

▲ Incentive Spirometer

▲ Oxygen

▲ Pulse Oximetry

▲ Suction Machines

▲ Tracheostomy

▲ Ventilators

THE DIGESTIVE SYSTEM

▲ Feeding Tubes

▲ Nasogastric Tubes

▲ Total Parenteral Nutrition (TPN)

▲ Colostomies

THE RENAL SYSTEM

▲ Bladder Scanner

▲ Catheters

▲ Continuous Bladder Irrigation (CBI)

▲ Ostomies

▲ Urine Collectors

THE MUSCULOSKELETAL SYSTEM

▲ Casts

▲ Drains

▲ Halo and Tongs

THE MUSCULOSKELETAL SYSTEM (CONT'D)

▲ Restraints

▲ Sutures (Stitches) and Staples

▲ Wheelchairs, Walkers, Crutches, Sliding Boards, and Beds

THE NEUROLOGICAL SYSTEM

▲ Lumbar Puncture (Spinal Tap)

THE METABOLIC SYSTEM

▲ Blood Glucose Monitoring

▲ Dialysis

PAIN CONTROL

▲ Patient-controlled Analgesia (PCA)

▲ Transcutaneous Electrical Nerve Stimulation (TENS)

THE CARDIOVASCULAR SYSTEM

BLOOD PRESSURE CUFF (SPHYGMOMANOMETER) AND STETHOSCOPE

This equipment monitors blood pressure, an important indicator of the functioning of the heart and blood vessels. High blood pressure can lead to strokes, kidney damage, and other damage to vital organs. Blood pressure is the force exerted on the inner walls of the arteries as blood flows through them. Blood pressure fluctuates constantly and rises with age, weight gain, stress, and emotions. It is

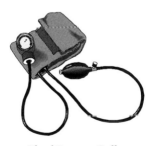

Blood Pressure Cuff

measured as millimeters of mercury rising in a gauge. Blood pressure is expressed as two numbers, the upper (systolic) and the lower (diastolic). The systolic number represents the maximum pressure on the arteries, which occurs when the left ventricle of the heart contracts. The diastolic number represents the minimum pressure on the arteries, which occurs during left ventricle relaxation. Blood pressure measurement indicates the state of the arteries themselves, whether they are narrowed and rigid or elastic and healthy.

The blood pressure cuff is inflatable and attached to a manual air pump and mercury gauge, which can be either mounted on the wall or portable. When the cuff is pumped up to the point at which the mercury reads at least 160, it stops arterial blood flow. The stethoscope's bell-shaped or flat, disk-shaped diaphragm is placed over a pulse point where blood flow can be heard easily, usually in the inner elbow. The sound is amplified through rubber tubes leading to earpieces. The cuff is slowly deflated and a first beat or "tap" is heard. This indicates the systolic pressure. The nurse notes the level of mercury on the numbered gauge when this occurs. Usually a series of five sounds is heard, the final one indicating the diastolic pressure. The nurse also notes where the mercury reading is when that happens. In a healthy person, the systolic pressure is usually between 140 and 100, the diastolic pressure between 90 and 60. The reading 120/80 is often used as a typical normal reading, but average blood pressure for a given individual could be 116/76 or 130/88. A systolic pressure consistently over 140 or diastolic pressure over 90 are cause for concern, however.

BLOOD TRANSFUSION

Blood is transfused into a vein or central line the same way as any other IV fluid. Whole blood, or separate components of blood such as packed red cells or plasma, may be given. A unit of blood is between 250 ml and 500 ml (about a cup to a pint), depending on what form of blood is being given. A patient may receive from one to many units.

An IV tubing called "Y-tubing" and an #18 or #20 gauge needle are used. The tubing forks into a Y at the top so that a bag of saline can be attached to one fork and the blood to the other. Saline solution is flushed through the tubing before the blood starts. Often a small filter is attached just below the unit of blood to ensure consistency of the fluid and a smoother flow. IV pumps are not generally used in blood transfusions.

Two nurses double-check the patient's identity and the blood product ordered before they hang the blood on the IV pole. They take the patient's vital signs just before the blood is started and fifteen minutes after to ensure that she/he does not have a reaction to the transfusion, signaled by fever, a fast pulse, or rapid breathing. Usually the patient does not feel anything at all unusual when receiving blood.

A unit of blood takes two to three hours to run through, although it may be given at a faster rate in an emergency or during surgery. Once the blood is finished, the tubing can be disconnected. If the patient had an IV solution running it can be reconnected. Medication is never added to blood.

CENTRAL LINE

A central line is a sterile catheter—a catheter is simply tubing that is usually larger than IV tubing—inserted into a large vein. The subclavian vein in the upper chest and the jugular vein in the neck are most often used. It is placed in those locations for two primary reasons:

▲ Poor veins in the arms and hands

▲ Large amounts of IV fluids needed for a long time

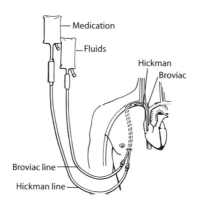

Central Line with Double Lumen

The central line can be inserted under a local anesthetic. Once sutured in place, the entry site is covered with a small dressing that is changed often. There are a variety of central lines. Some branch into two or three ends, called "lumen." Each lumen has a rubberized top that an IV needle can be plugged into. Each lumen is flushed with saline or heparin at regular intervals to make sure it is functioning well. Depending on the type of central line, this could be from every few hours to once a week.

CRASH CART

A "crash cart" is a waist-high metal cabinet on wheels with several drawers. It is a standard piece of equipment on hospital units. It is kept stocked with drugs and equipment used in emergency response to when a patient's heart stops beating.

Each of the crash cart's drawers holds specific items. One drawer has airway tubes, suction equipment, local anesthetic, and

---

CODED EMERGENCY ANNOUNCEMENTS

Every hospital has a set of coded emergency announcements that can be broadcast over the public address system to alert the staff without alarming the patients or visitors. These codes vary from hospital to hospital. For instance, "Red signal, fourth floor lounge" might indicate a fire in that location. Fires, flooding, and other unforeseen events do occur in hospitals. The code for a patient whose heart has stopped is often "Dr. Leo" or "code blue," followed by the room number. Unless there is a "Do Not Resuscitate" (DNR) order on a patient's chart or a "No Leo" indicated, the staff must respond promptly.

The staff member present when a cardiac arrest occurs immediately shouts to another staff member or calls the nurses' station and starts CPR (cardiopulmonary resuscitation). All professional staff are trained in CPR. Other staff rush the crash cart to the patient and members of the "Code Team" come running from other parts of the hospital. These usually include emergency room nurses and doctors.

laryngoscopes, instruments used to establish an airway in an unconscious patient. Another drawer has oxygen masks and tubing. Another contains IV supplies such as needles, tubing, and bags of IV solution, while yet another contains emergency drugs. These include atropine, epinephrine (adrenaline), sodium bicarbonate, and other drugs used to stimulate cardiac and respiratory functioning. As soon as the cart has been depleted, it is replaced or restocked. The items on it are checked by the nurses each night and tracked on lists kept on an attached clipboard.

DEFIBRILLATORS

Defibrillators are paddles that send an electric current through the heart. Two conduction pads are placed on the patient's chest and the paddles placed over them. Some varieties are placed on the chest and under the body. Defibrillators are used when a patient has ventricular fibrillation, an out-of-control pulsing of the heart's ventricles, or ventricular tachycardia, a very rapid heartbeat. The defibrillator current causes the heart muscle to normalize and resume its normal rhythm.

Newer automatic external defibrillators have a microcomputer that analyzes the heart rhythm. By visual or voice message it tells the operator when to push the button to activate the electric current. It then normalizes the conduction system in the heart and automatically reanalyzes its rhythm.

A bystander who accidentally touches a patient getting defibrillation can receive a shock.

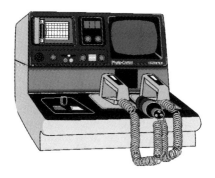

Defibrillator

ELECTROCARDIOGRAM (EKG OR ECG)

An electrocardiogram measures the electrical activity of the heart and shows it in the form of waves. Up to twelve electrodes, to which conducting gel has been applied, are placed on the arms, legs, and chest. An EKG can pinpoint disturbances in the heart's conduction and rhythm. These are caused by blockages in the heart's circulation, lack of oxygen to the heart muscle, or changes in the heart's electrochemical balance. Variations of the standard EKG are stress tests that measure the heart's activity when the patient is on a treadmill or bicycle. Holter monitors record heart performance and can be worn while the patient goes about his or her daily activities.

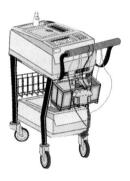

Electrocardiogram

IMPLANTED CATHETER

These devices can be implanted under the skin and left in place for up to a year. They consist of a small container, or reservoir, from which a small catheter leads to a vein. They form a slightly raised area under the skin that can be accessed by a needle. Implanted catheters function much like central lines but have no parts outside the body. They are often used to give chemotherapy, IV fluids, medication, and blood when such treatment is required for several months.

IMPLANTED IV LINES

Another option to deliver fluids to the arteriovascular system is a peripherally inserted central catheter line. A silicon or polyurethane flexible catheter with a single or double lumen, it is inserted

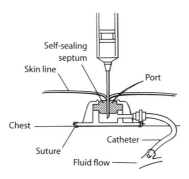

Implanted Catheter

into a vein in the arm and threaded through it into the superior vena cava or subclavian vein. It is sometimes used when a patient is getting IV therapy at home.

IV LINES

An IV is inserted into a vein to deliver fluid or medication directly into the bloodstream. An IV consists of a needle, tubing, and an IV bag or bottle. Most IV needles are actually fine plastic tubes. They are placed in the vein by a metal introducer needle that is then withdrawn, leaving the plastic needle, which is then taped in place.

To start an IV, a tourniquet is applied just above the vein that is to be used. If the vein is in the hand or forearm, the patient is asked to make a fist to help enlarge the vein. An effort is made to use the left hand in a right-handed person, but an IV can be inserted into almost any vein in the body, even in a foot if necessary. There is an unwritten rule that if, after three tries, a technician, nurse, or doctor cannot insert the needle, it's time to ask for someone else. IV needles and tubing are changed every three days.

Once the needle is in the vein, one end of the IV tubing screws into it while the other end pierces the seal on the IV bag with a plastic spike. A few inches down the tubing is the drip chamber, half-filled with the IV solution, where drops can be seen and counted. Further down the tubing is a simple roller clamp which is

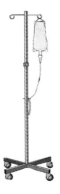

Intravenous Line

used to regulate the drip rate. Finally, the tubing has one or more sites to which additional IV lines can be attached by needle. These are small, sealed protuberances resembling twigs on a branch and are called "ports" or "Y-connector sites."

There are various kinds of IV tubing. Each manufacturer provides a built-in formula for the drip rate. If a patient is supposed to get 100 ml of IV solution per hour, one frequently used IV tubing is designed so that this works out to sixteen drops per minute. The nurse can adjust the rate by using the roller clamp on the tubing and timing the drops. In this case, there should be four drops every fifteen seconds, since there are sixteen drops per minute. There are many different IV solutions used, but they usually contain saline or glucose and water.

IV PUMPS

Electronic pumps are often used to regulate IV fluid delivery. These pumps are accurate and save time. The pump is attached to an IV pole and the tubing is threaded through the pump. Dials set the desired rate. The pump is plugged into an electrical outlet, but switches automatically to a battery should the power fail or the patient want to walk around pushing the IV pole. An alarm is activated if an air bubble develops or the line becomes kinked. The alarms are often over-sensitive. Problems can usually be fixed easily, in any case.

NEEDLES AND SYRINGES

Children run and strong men cringe at the sight of a needle, but it is one of the most effective ways to deliver medication to the body. The needles and syringes used now are almost all disposable, for one-time use only. Needles and plastic syringes are packaged separately. Once the needle and syringe are screwed together, the plastic cap on the needle is removed. A pull back on the syringe plunger draws liquid into the syringe. Any air bubbles are removed by flicking or tapping the sides of the syringe.

There are several diameter sizes of needles, from the relatively large #18 to the tiny #27. Different sizes are needed for the three basic types of injection:

▲ Intramuscular (IM)

▲ Subcutaneous (SQ)

▲ Intradermal

An IM injection is given into any large muscle, usually the upper buttock, upper arm, or thigh. The muscle is pulled taut and a #22 needle enters at a ninety-degree angle. Most pain medications and immunizations are given IM.

An SQ injection is given into a pinched fold of skin at a thirty-degree angle with a #25 needle. Examples of medications that are given SQ are heparin (a blood thinner) and insulin.

An intradermal injection is also given at a thirty-degree angle, just under the surface of the skin, with a #27 needle. Allergy shots are given this way.

Syringes also come in different sizes. The 3 ml syringe is used most often for injections. Some syringes hold only 1 ml and are

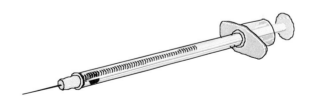

Syringe

then marked in fractions of that milliliter so that tiny amounts of medication can be given. Insulin syringes hold 1 ml and are divided into one hundred units to measure exact dosages, such as seventeen units.

Once used in the hospital, needle and syringe are dropped into special red biohazard containers attached to the walls in patients' rooms or near the nurses' station or medication room for later disposal.

SALINE LOCKS

Sometimes a patient may need an IV in order to receive an antibiotic or some other medication only every few hours, rather than a continuously running supply of fluid. In this case, a needle is inserted into a vein, filled with a tiny amount of saline solution or heparin (a blood thinner that prevents clotting), and simply capped with a rubber top. Later an IV needle and tubing can be inserted through the rubber top when needed. These are called "saline locks" or "heparin locks" and are flushed with saline or heparin every few hours to ensure that they remain clear. Flushing simply means injecting a small amount of solution and then withdrawing it.

SECONDARY IV LINES

Sometimes a second IV line is used to add other medication at set times. For instance, a patient may have a saline solution running into a vein, but may also need an antibiotic every six hours. Added medications usually come premixed in smaller bags with directions on how fast they are to run. The secondary medication IV, called a "piggyback," is connected to the main IV line with tubing and needle through a "port" and takes priority.

The secondary medication is usually delivered at a faster rate, so the IV pump is reprogrammed accordingly for the twenty minutes to an hour that the medication will probably run. Perhaps the main IV is going at 100 ml an hour, but the antibiotic is supposed to run at 150 ml an hour. It comes in a small 100 ml bag, so at a rate of 150 ml an hour it will run through in forty minutes. The pump is reset to 150 ml. The secondary medication bag is hung higher on the IV pole than the main IV, so gravity ensures that it will run instead. When it is finished, it is stopped by closing the roller clamp or "unplugging" its line and needle from the port in the main IV line. The nurse then reprograms the pump to 100 ml and the main IV resumes.

TELEMETRY

Sometimes a patient's heart activity is monitored continuously for several hours or days. There are various kinds of cardiac monitors. In telemetry, three electrodes are placed on the chest and attached by wires to a battery-powered transmitter worn next to the body. A Holter monitor is similar but self-contained in a pouch that allows the patient to go about his or her usual activities at home or work. The transmitter sends electrical signals to a monitor screen. On a cardiac unit, there may be several monitors placed near the nurses' station where they can be observed. An alarm rings if the heart rate rises or drops beyond certain limits.

THE RESPIRATORY SYSTEM

AIRWAY TUBES

An airway tube is a soft tube inserted through the nose or mouth to maintain an open passage for breathing when a patient is unconscious. (In a conscious patient, tube insertion could cause vomiting or muscle spasm.) An airway tube inserted through the nose is a rubber or latex tube. An airway tube inserted through the mouth is curved plastic or rubber. Airway tubes come in different lengths. The length is selected by measuring the distance between the tip of the nose and the earlobe. If you have an airway tube, you will be temporarily unable to speak.

An endotracheal tube is inserted orally or nasally beyond the vocal cords and into the trachea to facilitate mechanical ventilation. If you are conscious, local anesthetic is used. Endotracheal tubes are used after respiratory or cardiac arrest, when you stop breathing or your heart stops beating, or before surgery. The lubricated tube is guided by a tool called a laryngoscope, which is equipped with a light at the end. The tube also has a cuff that is inflated with 10 ml of air. Once the laryngoscope is removed, an X-ray is taken to ensure the tube's position. The tube is held in place with tapes or ties.

CHEST TUBES

Chest tubes are inserted into the pleural cavity, the space around the lungs, between two ribs. Chest tubes allow the drainage of excess air or fluid and permit a collapsed lung to expand. The chest tube is sutured in place and then connected to tubing from a drainage bottle. The connected section is reinforced with tape. A portable chest X-ray is done to check for correct position. Rubber-tipped clamps are placed at the bedside in case the tube becomes disconnected. A chest tube is usually left in place for a few days. The drainage system usually consists of one to three connected bottles that set up a closed-seal system. Sometimes a disposable plastic drainage apparatus is used.

INCENTIVE SPIROMETER

Sometimes a device called an incentive spirometer is used to improve breathing and lung capacity. Deep breathing exercises using the spirometer help to prevent pneumonia after surgery. A plastic cone several inches high, it has a tube the patient blows into. The goal is to make a small ball rise in the cone.

OXYGEN

If you are short of breath or have certain respiratory or heart conditions, you may need oxygen. Oxygen is delivered from units in the wall or small portable tanks on wheels. The amount of oxygen is measured in liters per minute and usually ranges from two liters to six or more. There are many kinds of oxygen masks. The simplest is tubing that loops around the ears and under the chin. Two small prongs emerge from the tube to fit into the nostrils. These are called nasal cannula. One or two liters of oxygen per minute can be delivered through them.

Other masks allow the patient to receive larger amounts of oxygen. A simple mask fits over the nose and mouth. Oxygen flows through tubing attached to an entry port at the bottom of the mask and out through two holes on the sides of the mask. A partial "rebreather" mask delivers a higher concentration of oxygen as you rebreathe some of the oxygenated air you exhale.

Continuous positive airway pressure (CPAP) supplies oxygen delivered under more pressure. It is used if you are already breathing on your own, but need more help or momentarily stop breathing while asleep, a condition called "sleep apnea." Oxygen levels in the blood are checked by testing arterial blood gases in blood samples, oximetry (see below), and observation of your color and breathing.

PULSE OXIMETRY

An oximeter is a machine that monitors the amount of oxygen in your arterial blood. Because there are numerous blood vessels in the fingers, a finger is placed in a holder called a photodetector. This is a type of transducer, or device that converts one kind of energy or information into another. Red or infrared light is sent through the finger and measured as it passes through the blood vessels. By measuring the absorption of light waves, the transducer detects the amount of color absorbed by the arterial blood and calculates the oxygen saturation. If it is outside normal limits, an alarm sounds. Oxygen saturation, ideally over 92%, appears as a number on a small screen. The patient is given oxygen if the saturation level is too low.

SUCTION MACHINE

Suctioning is the removal of excess fluids from the trachea and bronchi by inserting a thin tube called a suction catheter through the nose, mouth, airway tube, or tracheostomy tube. A suction machine with a pressure gauge and tubing is either attached to the wall or portable. The fluids sucked out enter a sealed drainage bottle.

The gauge is set at 80 to 120 mm of mercury. Saline solution is first sucked through the suction catheter to clean it and facilitate the procedure. There is a small opening on the side of the catheter, near the open tip. After the catheter is inserted, the nurse places a finger over this opening to increase the suction. The catheter is gently rotated for five seconds at a time.

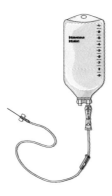

Suction Machine

TRACHEOSTOMY

A tracheostomy is a tube inserted into an opening made into the trachea from the neck. The procedure itself is called a "tracheotomy." A tracheostomy maintains an airway when the larynx is obstructed by swelling, blockage from a foreign body, tumor, or trauma. It can be temporary or permanent.

Tracheostomy tubes are metal or plastic, the latter having adaptors that enable them to be attached to ventilators if necessary. Some plastic tubes have a cuff that is inflated with 5 ml to 10 ml of air to give them a tighter seal. Other plastic tubes have caps that close up the opening and permit speech.

Most tracheostomy tubes have an outer and an inner tube. The inner tube (cannula) clicks or locks into the outer cannula. The tube can be disposable. If nondisposable, it is removed, cleaned with saline solution and sterile pipe cleaners, and replaced every shift. A tracheostomy tube has loops on each side that permit it to be tied around the neck with cotton tapes. Oxygen and suctioning equipment are kept at the bedside in case of emergency.

VENTILATORS

Mechanical ventilators, or respirators, move air in and out of your lungs when you are unable to do it on your own. Some ventilators deliver a preset amount of air each time. Others exert a positive pressure on the airway, forcing you to breathe in. Still others exert negative pressure that pulls the chest outward, allowing air to flow into the lungs.

Ventilator air temperature is regulated by a thermometer. To facilitate breathing, a patient on a ventilator is kept sitting semi-upright if possible, or turned from side to side at intervals. The amount of air delivered each time is called the "tidal volume." You can be gradually taken off, or "weaned," from the ventilator by decreasing the tidal volume and frequency of the breaths you are getting. You first must be able to breathe spontaneously at an adequate rate and strength.

THE DIGESTIVE SYSTEM

FEEDING TUBES

If you lack the ability to swallow due to a stroke, trauma, or paralysis, a feeding tube can be inserted into the stomach. One type of tube, a Dobbhoff, is passed through a nostril, down through the pharynx, and into the esophagus and stomach. The tubing is coated in lubricant and dipped in ice water first. You are placed sitting up at a ninety-degree angle and asked to sip ice water through a straw to ease the process. A fine guide wire inside the tube helps position the tube.

The tube is securely taped to the bridge of the nose and an X-ray is done to ensure proper placement. If placement is correct, the guide wire is slowly pulled out. The nurse can also check placement by injecting 50 ml of air by syringe into the tube and placing a stethoscope over the stomach to listen for the popping sound as the air passes through a muscle that guards the entrance to the stomach and enters the stomach. Removal of the tube when it is no longer needed simply involves withdrawing it gently.

Another kind of tube can be inserted through the abdominal wall directly into the stomach. This is called a percutaneous endoscopic gastrostomy (PEG) tube. It is easier to manage and clogs less than a tube inserted through the nose but involves surgery. Under anesthetic, it is inserted through a small incision in the stomach and sutured in place. A few inches long, the PEG has an attached cap to close it off. After twenty-four hours, small amounts of fluid are added to it at first. With this kind of tube, you can be given two- to three-cup feedings of liquid food (bolus feeds) every few hours by syringe or feeding pump.

Various feeding solutions, such as Ensure, Jevity, and Glucerna, can be prescribed by the doctor. For continuous feeding, a special pump the size of a small plastic box is attached to an IV pole. A quart-sized plastic bag or container is filled with fluid. It flows into tubing that is threaded through the pump and then connected to the end of the feeding tube. The pump is dialed to the desired rate and runs on electricity with battery backup. More fluid can be added to the top of the bag, and the tubing can also be disconnected at any time. If you are on tube feeding, you get medication through the tube, either in liquid form or as pills crushed in a small amount of water and given by syringe.

Tubes are flushed regularly with water to keep them open (patent). Warm water and cranberry juice are especially helpful in clearing narrower, nasally inserted tubes if they become blocked. If you are getting bolus feeds every few hours, a large syringe is used to gently draw back from the PEG tube before each bolus to see if there is an excess amount of fluid remaining in the stomach. This undigested amount is called the "residual." If it is more than 50 ml or so, the feeding is postponed until the stomach empties more. Residuals are also checked in patients on continuous feeding.

Often stroke patients are started on small amounts of soft or pureed food to test swallowing ability while still being tube fed. Tubes are easily removed if you regain the ability to swallow. Once a PEG tube is removed, the incision heals over.

NASOGASTRIC (NG) TUBES

Nasogastric tubes have many purposes. They can decompress the stomach after certain kinds of surgery. They are also used to wash out the stomach, obtain gastric fluids for analysis, prevent nausea, and provide feeding. Lubricated for easy insertion, NG tubes have a marker or strip near the end so that an X-ray can verify correct placement. Some have one passage, or lumen, others have two. A second lumen allows air to enter, which lets the tube float freely, rather than potentially irritating the stomach lining by sticking to it.

Some tubes go beyond the stomach and enter the intestinal tract. In these tubes, a balloon or rubber ring at the end holds water, air, or mercury to help the tube to pass and stimulate the normal peristaltic action of the digestive system's muscles. There are also tubes that are used to treat bleeding from the esophagus or stomach. They have inflatable balloons along the sides that exert pressure to control the bleeding.

Intestinal tubes are often attached to drainage suction pumps that exert mild pressure and pull excess contents into a drainage bottle. These drainage machines are either portable or attached to the wall. Close attention is paid to the amount and color of any drainage.

TOTAL PARENTERAL NUTRITION (TPN)

TPN is a method of giving special feeding liquids into a vein. It supplies all the body's nutritional needs. TPN is used when you are nutritionally at risk but, for a variety of reasons, unable to take food by mouth or through a feeding tube. A catheter is inserted through a large vein, usually the superior vena cava in the upper chest. The catheter is usually left in place for at least two weeks. It contains special filters and the tubing attached to it is changed every three days. The feeding solution, prepared in the hospital pharmacy according to the doctor's orders, is absorbed into the body through the bloodstream. IV fluids, blood, or medications are never added to TPN. The feeding bottle or bag hangs on an IV pole and drips at the rate ordered.

COLOSTOMIES

After some kinds of surgeries, a patient may be left with a temporary or permanent opening from the large intestine called a

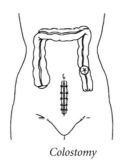

Colostomy

colostomy. An external disposable pouch collects emptying fecal matter from the opening. Like the ileostomy products described on page 92, there are many different colostomy products available.

THE RENAL SYSTEM

BLADDER SCANNER

If the doctor thinks the bladder is not emptying completely, a bladder scan can be done right after you void to see how much urine, if any, remains in the bladder. A bladder that does not empty fully can allow infection to develop. A bladder scanner is a small ultrasound device. When lubricated with conducting gel and placed over the lower abdomen, it gives a printout of the volume of urine in the bladder.

CATHETERS

A catheter is a soft, flexible tube of narrow diameter used to drain fluid from an organ. It is most often used to drain urine from the bladder when it is unable to empty normally due to injury, infection, muscle spasm, paralysis, or lack of muscle tone.

"In and out" catheterization may be done just once or every few hours. A catheter may also be left in place days, weeks, months, or semipermanently. It is changed about every three weeks. In an "in and out" procedure, a straight catheter a few inches long is inserted through the opening of the urethra and into the bladder until urine starts to drain out. It is virtually painless for most females, but may be slightly uncomfortable for males unless a topical anesthetic ointment or cream is used. It is a sterile procedure, which means that the skin area is cleaned first and the nurse wears sterile gloves. The catheters are packaged in sterile containers. They are lubricated and come with a small container into which the urine drains.

If a catheter is to stay in place for a while, a Foley catheter is used. It has an inflatable balloon that sits just inside the neck of the bladder, anchoring it in place. There are two inner passages, or "lumen," in the tube—one to drain the urine and the other to inflate the balloon. To inflate it, a syringe containing 10 ml to 15 ml of sterile water is inserted into the closed end of the section leading to the balloon. To remove the catheter, a needle and syringe is inserted and the plunger drawn back to pull the water out, deflating the balloon. The catheter then slides out. The catheter is attached by tubing to a drainage bag that is emptied every eight hours. It should hang on the bottom of the bed frame to allow gravity to help urine drain. There are also leg bags that can be attached by straps and are invisible under long pants.

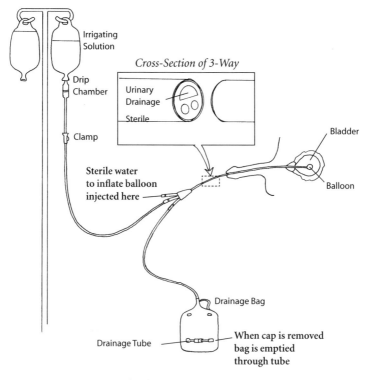

Continuous Bladder Irrigation with 3-Way Catheter

CONTINUOUS BLADDER IRRIGATION (CBI)

Sometimes it is desirable to continually rinse a fluid through the bladder to help the bladder heal, especially after prostate and other surgery. This is called "continuous bladder irrigation." Saline solutions in three-quart bags are often used. Three-way catheters, with three lumen, are used for CBI: one to drain the urine, one to inflate the balloon, and one to run the irrigating solution into. The irrigating solution bags hang on IV poles and the flow rate is regulated by clamps. The goal is to keep the urine clear in color and the flow rate is adjusted accordingly. This fluid drains out through the same lumen as the urine. A running account is kept of how much solution goes in and this amount is subtracted from the total output in the drainage bag in order to get the true volume of urine.

OSTOMIES

After various kinds of surgery or trauma, provisions can be made to drain urine directly from openings in the urinary system. A tube placed directly into the bladder is called a cystostomy tube or suprapubic catheter. A nephrostomy tube drains from a kidney. These are often temporary. More permanent openings, called "stoma," are made in the ureters or upper intestine and called ureterostomies, ileal conduits, or urinary diversions.

There are many products on the market for use with these openings. A skin barrier cream is usually applied around the opening and a square, flat wafer with a sticky backing is cut to fit the opening. It is pressed gently against the skin and connected to a drainage bag or pouch. A raised plastic ring on the wafer patch clicks onto a matching ring on the bag. The bag has an opening on the bottom to drain it, with a plastic clamp to close it.

Bags should be emptied when a third to a half full. They can be reused if washed, and at night can be connected by tubing to a drainage bag. Similar bags are used after bowel surgery when the contents of the intestines must empty through a colostomy. Hospitals usually have educational information packets and nurse clinicians or resource people to teach you how to manage these devices.

URINE COLLECTORS

When you have a catheter, urine is measured from the drainage bag every eight hours. But sometimes patients without catheters are asked to save their urine in a container that fits inside the toilet. The amount of fluid you drink, plus any IV fluid you get, is also measured. You are said to be on "in and out." More fluid should go in than comes out in order to maintain a positive fluid balance in the body and prevent dehydration.

Sometimes a twenty-four hour urine collection is needed to test components in the urine. It is started in the morning. You discard the first void of the day and then save the rest, pouring it into a special container, which may have certain preservatives added. If it is suspected that you have kidney stones (renal calculi), you may be asked to strain your urine through a screened container to catch any stone fragments for analysis.

THE MUSCULOSKELETAL SYSTEM

CASTS

Casts immobilize and protect body parts, usually fractured bones. They are made of plaster, fiberglass, or other materials. Plaster casts are applied wet. They take several hours to dry and feel slightly warm while doing so. Fiberglass casts are lighter. It is important to make sure the cast is not too tight by checking the color, sensation, and movement in fingers and toes and to watch for any swelling. Casts are removed easily with a cutting wheel or saw applied along one side. You usually feel some heat and vibration. A tongs-like spreader then opens the cut wider and scissors finish the job, cutting padding underneath. The arm, leg, or body part exposed is usually pale, dry, and scaly.

Traction exerts a pulling action to align fractures, treat dislocations, or decrease muscle spasm. A pulley and weight provides a counterforce. The two main types are skin traction and skeletal traction. Skin traction exerts a lighter pull on padding attached to an arm or leg. It is used most often on legs and feet. In skeletal traction, a pin or wire is inserted through the bone and then attached to the traction equipment. Frames and triangular forms hanging over the bed (called "trapezes") allow you to move more easily and lift yourself off the bed.

DRAINS

After orthopedic or other surgery, a wound may have a drainage tube placed in it temporarily. This assists in removing excess fluids to promote healing. A drain may be only an inch or two in length and held in place by a suture.

HALO AND TONGS

Sometimes a halo is used to align the head and neck after injury to the neck vertebrae. A metal ring fits around the head and bars connect the halo to a hard plastic vest lined with sheepskin. There are several sizes and they can be adjusted. Four pin sites are chosen, and under local anesthetic, pins are screwed into the skull at ninety-degree angles and attached to the headband by wires.

Another form of traction, called tongs, consists of wires attached to pins on both sides of the skull. When you are lying flat, the wires exert a gentle pull because they are attached to a half-circle of metal placed above the head and connected to a traction frame.

RESTRAINTS

Unfortunately, there are times when a patient must be placed in wrist restraints or a jacket called a "Posey vest." This is a last resort, used only when other measures have failed. For instance, the patient may need an IV or Foley catheter but, due to an inability to comprehend reminders, may keep pulling at the tubing. An elderly, disoriented patient, a severely brain-injured patient, or someone with a violent reaction to a street drug may cause injury to herself/himself and prevent treatment unless she/he is restrained. The doctor may write a restraint order in such cases.

Restraint policies vary among hospitals, but an order is usually limited to only a few hours and then must be renewed. Sometimes an order is continually renewed for several days. The reason for the use of restraints must be thoroughly documented in the nurses' notes and on special forms.

Wrist restraints are soft cloth or sheepskin cuffs with long ties that are fastened to the bottom of the bed frame. A Posey vest is a cloth vest that zips up the back and also has ties. It is not the same as a straightjacket. Special slip knots are used so they can be untied quickly. A patient in restraints must be repositioned, turned, checked on often, and have all her/his nutritional and toileting needs met.

SUTURES (STITCHES) AND STAPLES

Sutures are used to close an incision or tear, or to hold tubes in place. Local anesthetic is usually sprayed or injected at the site if you are conscious. Various thicknesses of fine nylon thread are used in many different stitching patterns. They may be removed about a week later, though some dissolve over time.

Sometimes metal staples are used to close large incisions. When the wound has healed, they are easily removed by a nurse with extractor clippers. Tiny adhesive strips, called "steri strips," can be placed at intervals over the incisions for a few more days.

WHEELCHAIRS, WALKERS, CRUTCHES, SLIDING BOARDS, AND BEDS

There are dozens of wheelchair designs, ranging from basic styles to electric models that cost as much as a Mercedes. Footrests and arms are usually removable and/or adjustable. All-important are the brakes, which should be locked before anyone gets into or out of a wheelchair.

Walkers provide stability and security when walking is unsteady. They come in different sizes and heights and usually fold up when not in use. "Quad canes" that have a steadying base made up of four splayed legs also provide stability.

Crutches come in different heights. Be sure to ask about the techniques involved in using them, including how to go up and down stairs.

A sliding board is a smooth board about two feet by eight inches in size, with a nonstick surface on the bottom. Wedged under a buttock, the board allows you to slide from a wheelchair placed alongside a bed to the bed, with minimal or no help.

The head and foot of a hospital bed can be adjusted up or down by pushing a button on the bed rail. There are also controls at the foot of the bed. If you are bedridden, special beds and mattresses reduce pressure on the skin. They work much like water beds.

THE NEUROLOGICAL SYSTEM

LUMBAR PUNCTURE (SPINAL TAP)

A lumbar puncture is the insertion of a sterile needle into the space around the spinal cord, usually in the lower spine. It is done for the following reasons:

▲ To obtain specimens of cerebrospinal fluid, which bathes the brain and spinal cord.

▲ To measure intercranial pressure.

▲ To inject dyes used in X-rays of the brain and spinal cord.

▲ To give some forms of anesthesia.

Local anesthetic is used first and the needle and syringe are attached to a three-way stopcock and a manometer, which is a pressure gauge used, in this case, to measure intercranial pressure.

THE METABOLIC SYSTEM

BLOOD GLUCOSE MONITORING

It is important for patients who have diabetes to check their blood sugar. Blood glucose levels that are too high or too low can cause a variety of complications ranging from feeling faint to circulatory problems to coma. Depending on the severity of the disease, blood glucose is checked anywhere from occasionally to four times a day, before each meal and at bedtime. There are a number of machines on the market that make such testing quick and easy. Most involve pricking a finger to get a drop of blood, placing the drop on a slide or test strip, and putting the strip into the machine to get a reading. Some machines are as small as a pocket calculator.

Diabetes occurs when the pancreas produces insufficient insulin to control and balance the amount of sugar in the body. Blood levels of sugar are checked in the hospital so that you can be given insulin if the blood sugar is too high. The doctor orders insulin on an individual basis for each patient. It is important that you learn how to monitor blood sugar at home and notify the doctor of unexpected changes.

DIALYSIS

Basically, dialysis takes over the work of nonfunctioning kidneys. Dialysis can be done through a blood vessel in the arm, which is called "hemodialysis," or through the abdomen, called "peritoneal dialysis." Dialysis is usually carried out three times per week and takes several hours each time. Using the principle that matter moves from an area of high concentration to low concentration, a special membrane allows fresh solution to pass into the bloodstream and draws away toxic wastes.

In hemodialysis, blood is taken from the body, circulated through a purifying dialyzer liquid, and then returned to the body. An arteriovenous connection called a "fistula" is made in the arm. An artery and vein are sutured together, leaving a common opening an inch or so in length. A variation on this is called an "arteriovenous shunt," made when tubing connects the vein and artery in a small synthetic loop that extends just outside the skin. An "arteriovenous graft" is a similar connection.

In peritoneal dialysis, the exchange of fresh fluid and wastes occurs through a semipermanent catheter placed under the skin in the abdomen. Machines to which bags of dialyzing fluids are attached carry out the dialysis. Nurses who perform dialysis must be specially trained to do so. In some cases patients can be taught to self-dialyze at home using smaller, portable machines.

PAIN CONTROL

PATIENT-CONTROLLED ANESTHESIA (PCA)

PCA delivers pain-killing drugs (called "analgesics") to you. You have some control over the amount and rate of the drug given. Delivery of the drug can be continuous, with the ability to boost the intensity of the drug to a higher level yourself, or it can be programmed so that you can administer the drug sporadically, as needed. In the hospital, a computerized pump called a PCA pump is attached to an IV pole and a small cassette-like container of morphine or other drug is slipped into it. The medication reaches you through an IV line. Other devices for use at home are implanted under the skin or worn next to the body and connected by needle to a vein.

Obviously you must be mentally alert to use a PCA pump. The goal is to relieve pain but not overload you so that you become drowsy and unable to speak. PCA is used most often post-operatively and for terminally ill patients.

TRANSCUTANEOUS ELECTRICAL NERVE STIMULATION (TENS)

A TENS unit is a small battery-powered device that sends painless electric current over nerve pathways. This blocks your perception of pain by providing counteracting stimuli. The unit can be looped over a belt or worn under clothing. Four flexible wires attach the battery to electrodes that stick to the skin. TENS is usually used for several hours at a time for chronic or acute pain or after surgery. Correct placement of the electrodes is important in order to get maximum effect from the TENS unit. Dials control the current's strength; too low a setting is ineffective, while too high a setting can be uncomfortable. With experimentation and fine-tuning, you can benefit greatly from this device.

Drugs:
WHAT YOU DON'T KNOW
CAN HURT YOU

A s a patient, it's important for you to know what you're taking and why. Certain drugs taken in combination can have harmful side effects. Other drugs should be taken on an empty stomach or with food. Most drugs should also be taken at scheduled times.

There are thousands of drugs on the market today. Pharmaceutical company representatives constantly pitch new drugs to doctors. They leave free samples and offer incentives to prescribe their products. New and improved variations on long-established drugs are legion. Today's new wonder drug for high blood pressure may be replaced in six months by a rival medication. No wonder the list of drugs doctors frequently prescribe is in a state of flux. No doctor can possibly know everything about every drug. But most doctors have certain drugs they favor and others they dislike, based on trial-and-error experience.

GENERIC AND BRAND NAMES

Names of drugs can be confusing. Each drug has a generic name, based on the drug's chemical content. There may also be different brand names for a drug. For instance, the generic heart drug digoxin is often marketed under the trade name Lanoxin. A sulfa drug often used to treat urinary tract infections is sold as Bactrim, Septra, and several other brands.

PRESCRIBING DRUGS AT THE HOSPITAL

A doctor prescribes a drug for you by leaving either a written order in your chart or a telephone order with a nurse. The nurse signs the written order to show that she/he has seen it and notes the date and time with the signature. If the nurse has taken a verbal order, she/he writes it in the doctors' orders section of the chart, but the doctor must sign it later. The chart is then "flagged" or marked in some way to call the doctor's attention to it. A unit clerk sends a copy of the order to the hospital pharmacy, usually by fax. For reasons of clarity, the pharmacy should always get an order in written form. A verbal message can result in misunderstanding and error.

THE FORMULARY

Each hospital pharmacy carries a list of standard drugs referred to as the hospital's "formulary," or set list of drugs on hand. If a doctor orders a drug not listed on the formulary, the pharmacy may have to send out for it to another hospital or pharmacy or replace it with something else.

DELIVERING AND ADMINISTERING MEDICATIONS

Pharmacy technicians deliver drugs to hospital floors on regular rounds throughout the day. Each patient's medications are usually packaged and labeled separately and kept in a locked drawer or cupboard. On some units drugs are stored in cabinets accessed by computer codes. "Controlled" drugs, such as narcotics, sedatives, and sleeping pills, are locked up. Whenever a nurse takes one to you, she/he must fill out information on a narcotics sheet, including your name, the drug, the amount, the time, and the nurse's name. This keeps a running tally of the supply of each drug. At change of shift time, a nurse who is leaving and one who is coming on must count the controlled drugs to reconcile the amounts with the number signed out.

You may bring your own pills to the hospital, but you are usually required to surrender them for safekeeping. It's easiest to simply bring a list of your medications, because the doctor may change them during your hospital stay. If they remain unchanged or if, for reasons of cost, you want to use your own medications, they will be locked up and brought to you by a nurse. Insulting as this may seem, its rationale is the avoidance of confusion and duplication. The nurse is responsible for seeing you actually take the medication, since it is she/he who must sign it off on the medication sheet in your chart. The times at which you get your medication may also differ from your home routine. If a nurse is passing out 8:00 P.M. pills to eight patients, some will get them a little before 8:00 P.M. and some a little after.

TIPS FOR APPROPRIATE USE

There is no question that many drugs are overused. Individuals are often prescribed too many drugs at one time. If you are under the care of more than one doctor, you should make each one aware of the medications prescribed by the other. Interactions between drugs are not always fully understood or anticipated. What works for one person may not work for another. And the list of potential side effects of most drugs is truly daunting. For anyone susceptible to the power of suggestion, it's almost better not to read about the side effects in advance, but to simply take the prescribed drug, see how it goes, and hope for the best. This is not to say, however, that truly annoying side effects should not be reported to your doctor.

The elderly, in particular, need careful monitoring and assessment of their medications. Slower metabolisms cause drugs to clear your system more gradually and the potential for drug interaction is greater.

There are many guides to frequently used drugs for the lay person. A list of them appears in the "Resources" section at the back of this book. In the following section, frequently prescribed drugs are discussed under headings related to the major body systems. It is not meant to be a comprehensive discussion of drugs, but merely to inform you about some of the drugs commonly prescribed for patients in the hospital.

THE CARDIOVASCULAR SYSTEM

There are many drugs that treat problems of the cardiovascular system.

ANTIARRHYTHMICS

Drugs called antiarrhythmics help to establish a steady heart rhythm and stabilize the heart. These include drugs with the generic names procainamide, quinidine, and lidocaine hydrochloride, among others. In emergencies such as cardiac arrest, epinephrine is given intravenously and can even be injected into the heart muscle to restore cardiac rhythm when the heart has stopped.

ANTIHYPERTENSIVES

Drugs that treat high blood pressure (hypertension) are called antihypertensives. There are many varieties, some for long-term use and others for sudden, severe spikes in blood pressure.

▲ Nifedipine is marketed under such names as Procardia and Adalat. In emergencies, the capsule can be punctured with a needle and the liquid medication squeezed under the tongue.

▲ Some antihypertensives suppress the control centers in the brain that cause blood vessels to constrict. Catapres, for instance, lowers arterial resistance and relaxes blood vessels.

▲ Diuretics lower blood pressure by reducing sodium and water retention in the body.

▲ Beta blockers like propranolol (Inderal) and metoprolol (Lopressor) and calcium channel blockers, such as verapamil (Cardizem), lower blood pressure by keeping the artery walls from constricting. Dosages can be adjusted through consultation between you and your doctor. Potential side effects are similar to those seen in drugs used to treat angina and include light-headedness, dizziness, fatigue, and low blood pressure.

BLOOD THINNERS

Blood thinners prevent or treat heart attacks, inflammation of veins (phlebitis), and blood clots. Drugs such as streptokinase are sometimes used immediately after a heart attack as they contain enzymes that dissolve blockages in the heart's arteries. Heparin is given continuously by IV to dissolve clots. Your blood is tested regularly to determine whether it is losing its tendency to form clots. The amount and rate of heparin is adjusted accordingly.

Once the blood has thinned you can take an oral anticoagulant, such as Coumadin (warfarin sodium), in pill form. Coumadin inhibits the action of vitamin K, which is essential in clot formation. It should be taken at the same time every day. You should avoid taking aspirin, which also has some blood-thinning ability, and you should watch for unexpected bruises, bleeding gums, or nosebleeds. These could indicate that the level of blood thinner is too high, causing tiny hemorrhages.

Another product called Lovenox (enoxaparin sodium), a heparin derivative, is a blood thinner with few side effects. It is injected into the abdomen subcutaneously for seven to ten days following hip replacement surgery and has proven effective in preventing blood clots.

CHOLESTEROL-LOWERING DRUGS

Cholesterol, found in foods containing saturated fats and organ meats like liver and kidneys, causes plaque to build up and narrow the arteries. High cholesterol is usually due to genetic factors as well as a high-fat, high-cholesterol diet. This leaves you vulnerable to cardiovascular problems such as heart attacks and strokes. Besides dietary changes, certain medications can lower cholesterol. Several drugs have been developed to inhibit cholesterol production, including the generic drugs lovastatin and pravastatin sodium.

DIGOXIN

Digoxin slows and strengthens the heart muscle when it is not performing efficiently. It is used to treat congestive heart failure, where the heart is no longer able to pump an adequate supply of blood to meet the body's demand. Digoxin also effectively treats a too-rapid heartbeat (tachycardia) and atrial fibrillation, where the heart's upper chambers flutter in a disorganized and ineffectual pattern. Before taking digoxin, the pulse is checked each time for a full minute to make sure it is at least sixty beats per minute. If less than that, digoxin is not given, as it would slow the heart too much.

NITROGLYCERIN

For angina, the chest pain caused by blockages in major blood vessels that restrict blood flow to the heart muscle, the standard drug used is nitroglycerin. It helps to increase blood flow through smaller, secondary blood vessels. Nitroglycerin is most often given in the form of a tiny pill that melts under the tongue. It can be given up to three times, five minutes apart, until effective. If ineffective, you need emergency attention. Nitroglycerin is also available as a patch and as an ointment applied to a paper square that is taped in place. Both slowly release medication through the skin and are worn for several hours at a time. Possible side effects include light-headedness, dizziness, headache, and fatigue.

THE RESPIRATORY SYSTEM

Besides the antibiotics used to treat infections ranging from sinus conditions to pneumonia, respiratory system drugs include antihistamines and bronchodilators.

ANTIHISTAMINES

Antihistamines block the histamine production that causes runny nose, itching, and sneezing. They are marketed under many brand names. Diphenhydramine hydrochloride (Benadryl) reduces the above symptoms as well as suppressing motion sickness. Side effects of antihistamines may include drowsiness, dizziness, headache, and dryness of the mouth and throat. Antihistamines should not be combined with alcohol.

BRONCHODILATORS

Bronchodilators relax the smooth muscle of the bronchial tubes and pulmonary blood vessels. They provide relief if you suffer from asthma, emphysema, or chronic obstructive airway disease. Bronchodilators include theophylline (Aminophylline), albuterol (Proventil), and ipratropium bromide (Atrovent), among others. They are given as pills, through inhalers (in mist form through an oxygen mask), or by injection.

EPINEPHRINE

When the throat closes due to anaphylactic shock caused by an extreme allergic reaction to a bee sting, medicine, or other substance, epinephrine, also called adrenaline, brings fast relief when given as an injection.

THE DIGESTIVE SYSTEM

ANTACIDS

The most frequently used digestive system drugs are common antacids such as aluminum hydroxide and magnesium hydroxide found in such products as Maalox and Mylanta.

ANTINAUSEA DRUGS

Antinausea medications act on the brain to inhibit the vomiting response. Dimenhydrinate (Dramamine), for example, stops nausea and motion sickness. Possible side effects include drowsiness, dizziness, low blood pressure, and headache.

For the nausea and vomiting sometimes caused by cancer chemotherapy, tetrahydrocannabinol (Marinol), the main ingredient in marijuana, may be prescribed. Other drugs effective against nausea include phenergan, ondansetron, and prochlorperazine. Many of these drugs can be administered by injection or intravenously.

ANTIULCER DRUGS

Some drugs focus on healing ulcers of the stomach and duodenum, the upper part of the small intestine. Ulcers are areas in the lining of these organs that have been worn away. Bacteria also play a role in causing ulcers; therefore, antibiotics are often part of the cure. Other drugs decrease gastric acid production. They contain cimetidine and other ingredients. Another medication, sucralfate (Carafate), forms a protective barrier over the ulcer.

THE RENAL SYSTEM

DIURETICS

Diuretics rid the body of excess fluids by increasing the kidneys' output. They are sometimes called "water pills." Diuretics are used to treat buildup of fluids in the lungs (pulmonary edema), generalized swelling (edema), high blood pressure, and acute or chronic renal failure. Furosemide (Lasix) is probably the most frequently prescribed diuretic, but there are many others, such as hydrochlorthiazide (Hydrudiuril). Furosemide can be given as a pill or injected into IV tubing. A daily dose should be taken in the morning since an evening dose will result in sleep interrupted by trips to the bathroom.

The side effects of diuretics like furosemide may include low blood pressure, dizziness, abdominal pain, ringing in the ears, dehydration, and low levels of sodium and potassium, electrolytes that help regulate the heart's rhythm. Anyone taking a diuretic should take a potassium supplement or eat a high-potassium diet. Bananas, citrus fruit, and tomatoes are rich sources of potassium. Periodic blood tests for electrolyte levels and kidney functioning (BUN) should be given. Patients taking digoxin should have periodic blood tests to measure digoxin levels, which can be affected by diuretics.

THE MUSCULOSKELETAL SYSTEM

Some drugs are prescribed to reduce muscle spasticity in patients affected by multiple sclerosis and certain spinal cord injuries. One of them is baclofen (Lioresal) and given as a pill or by intravenous pump. Drugs such as alendronate sodium (Fosamax) increase the formation of calcium. Erythropoietin (Epogen) stimulates the rate of red blood cell formation in the bone marrow.

THE NEUROLOGICAL SYSTEM

It is easy to understand how medications that produce physical changes in the body work. Antibiotics clear up infections. Diuretics remove excess fluid from the body. Nitroglycerin reduces chest pain caused by sluggish blood flow to the heart. These drugs have somewhat more predictable effects—and side effects—than drugs that act on the mind and emotions.

ANTIANXIETY DRUGS

Coping with illness, dealing with surgery, and being in an unfamiliar place that is buzzing with activity can lead to anxiety and stress. In the hospital, drugs are sometimes prescribed to reduce anxiety and tension and to increase relaxation. After all, healing occurs more rapidly when the body is resting. Antianxiety drugs are also used to relax you before surgery and to help you sleep. Like many drugs, there is no question that they can be over-prescribed at times and have some negative side effects. But they have their place. They can effectively calm the agitation and irritability caused by dementia, for instance. Medication can calm the delirium caused by severe metabolic imbalances such as "thyroid storm," a rare thyroid disorder, or by other diseases like meningitis.

Mood altering drugs are popularly referred to as sedatives or tranquilizers, but these categories overlap. All of them depress the activity of the central nervous system and affect the limbic and subcortical levels of the brain. Some of the drugs used to calm patients are benzodiazepines. Their generic names usually end in "-pam," as in lorazepam (Ativan). Benzodiazepines fall into short-acting groups, which are cleared from the body in a few hours, and long-acting groups, whose effects may last twenty hours or more. Examples of short-acting benzodizepines are the sleeping pills oxazepam (Serax), temazepam (Restoril), and triazolam (Halcion).

Longer-acting benzodiazepines include the following:

▲ Clonazepam (Klonopin) and flurazepam hydrochloride (Dalmane)

▲ Chlordiazepoxide (Librium), also used in the treatment of alcohol withdrawal

▲ Diazepam (Valium), used as a muscle relaxant as well as an antianxiety drug

Many other non-benzodiazepines are available. Examples include the antianxiety drug buspirone hydrochloride (BuSpar) and the sleeping pill zolpidem tartrate (Ambien).

Another class of drugs, the barbiturates, produce stronger sedation. These end in the generic suffix "-al," as in pentobarbital (Nembutal) and secobarbital (Seconal).

Since all these drugs can cause dependence, they should be withdrawn slowly by tapering them off. They accumulate in the system, and the elderly, in particular, can build up excessive amounts, causing drowsiness or dizziness. Antianxiety drugs should not be combined with alcohol for the same reason. On rare occasions they can have the opposite effect from their intended purpose. Rather than calming you, they can cause loss of inhibition, euphoria, and wild excitement.

ANTICONVULSANTS

Other neurological drugs include anticonvulsants. These drugs control seizures caused by epilepsy, trauma to the head, or other neurological disorders. Examples include carbamazepine (Tegretol) and valproic acid (Depakane), as well as phenytoin (Dilantin) and clonazepam (Klonopin), a benzodiazepine with anticonvulsant effects.

NARCOTICS

Narcotics dull the senses, relieve pain, and can cause profound sleep, stupor, or coma. The heart rate and breathing slow down and the pupils are reduced in size, sometimes to pinpoints. Many of the narcotics used in hospitals are derived from synthetic opium.

The most commonly prescribed narcotic drugs are used for moderate to severe pain and include the following:

▲ Acetaminophen and codeine (Tylenol #2 and Tylenol #3)

▲ Propoxyphene hydrochloride (Darvon)

▲ Propoxyphene napsylate (Darvocet)

▲ Acetaminophen and oxycodone hydrochloride (Percocet)

▲ Acetaminophen and hydrocodone bitartrate (Lortab)

▲ Pentazocine (Talwin)

▲ Hydromorphone hydrochloride (Dilaudid)

Most of these drugs are taken in pill form, although some, such as Talwin, can be injected.

Meperidine hydrochloride (Demerol) is used for severe pain and usually given by intramuscular (IM) injection.

Morphine can be given in tablet form, IM, into an IV line, and continuously through a morphine pump. It is also available as a gradual-release pill and a skin patch.

PAIN MEDICATIONS

Drugs that reduce pain are called "analgesics" and act by interfering with pain receptors in the brain and neurological system.

Most analgesics relieve pain and reduce fever. Common nonnarcotic pain medications include:

▲ Acetaminophen (Tylenol and other brands).

▲ Acetylsalicylic acid (aspirin), which also has an anti-inflammatory effect and may prevent blood clots. However, if taken regularly, it can cause stomach bleeding in some susceptible people.

▲ Ibuprofen (Motrin), a nonsteroidal anti-inflammatory drug (NSAID) used to treat the symptoms of arthritis, gout, and menstrual cramps. Ibuprofen should be taken with food or milk.

THE METABOLIC SYSTEM

CORTICOSTEROIDS

Drugs that affect the body's metabolism include corticosteroids. They suppress the out-of-control immune system response that can cause healthy tissue to be mistakenly attacked by the body's immune system, as seen in rheumatoid arthritis. Corticosteroids suppress inflammation and are also used to treat exacerbations of multiple sclerosis. Prednisone is a corticosteroid. Another is dexamethasone (Decadron), used to relieve swelling of the brain, or cerebral edema. It can be given as a pill or intravenously. The side effects of corticosteroids may include weight gain, high blood pressure, and disturbances of the body's electrolyte balance. These are powerful drugs but different from the steroids used by athletes.

DIABETES DRUGS

One of the most common metabolic disorders is diabetes. It can occur in mild, moderate, or severe form. Diabetes is caused by a deficiency of insulin, a hormone secreted by the pancreas to regulate the use of sugar (glucose) in the body. It can also occur when the body is unable to use insulin properly. Diabetes can lead to many complications. These include circulatory problems, vulnerability to infection, and eye problems.

Along with diet, weight reduction, and exercise, medication often forms a part of a diabetes treatment plan. Oral medications help the body use insulin more effectively. These medications include glipizide (Glucotrol), glyburide (DiaBeta), and others.

Sometimes diabetes requires insulin injections, which are given subcutaneously since insulin is destroyed by stomach acids. There are many different kinds of insulin, categorized according to whether they are short-, medium-, or long-acting:

▲ Short-acting insulins (regular and semilente) are effective for up to eight hours.

▲ Medium-acting insulins (lente, NPH, and 70/30) act for up to twenty-four hours.

▲ Long-acting insulins (ultralente) can last for up to thirty-six hours.

The following should be kept in mind if you use insulin:

▲ It should be kept in a cool place and the expiration date checked.

▲ Blood sugar is checked from one to four times a day, and insulin levels are adjusted based on test results.

▲ Different types of insulin may be combined in one syringe. For example, you may take NPH insulin for your routine dosage but use regular insulin for any extra units needed.

THYROID MEDICATION

Another metabolic drug is levothyroxin sodium (Synthroid). When the thyroid gland is not functioning up to par, due to deficiencies of thyroid hormone, levothyroxin stimulates the thyroid and increases metabolism in all the body's tissues. Side effects may include tremors, nervousness, and rapid heartbeat. To maintain constant hormone levels, levothyroxin should be taken at the same time every day, usually in the morning.

THE IMMUNE SYSTEM

These drugs include corticosteroids such as prednisone (Delta-sone) that suppress the immune response and decrease inflammation. A number of side effects can occur, including stomach irritation, high blood pressure, and delayed healing of cuts. A drug called lymphocytic immune globulin is given to kidney transplant patients to prevent the body from rejecting the new organ. Vaccines contain tiny amounts of bacteria or viruses modified with other substances so that they are no longer dangerous but activate the build-up of an immune response in the body. Diptheria, tetanus, and hepatitis A and B are examples of diseases that can be prevented by vaccination.

DRUGS FREQUENTLY PRESCRIBED IN THE HOSPITAL

ANTIBIOTICS

Antibiotics destroy many common and dangerous bacteria and are grouped according to the specific bacteria they kill. They are not effective against viruses. Some can be taken by mouth, while others are most effective when injected or given intravenously. The best known of the antibiotics are the penicillins. There are many different penicillins, the names always ending in "-cillin," as in amoxicillin, ampicillin, and cloxacillin, for instance. Erythromycin is sometimes used to treat pelvic inflammatory disease and intestinal infections. Vancomycin, always given intravenously, fights severe staphylococcus infections for which other antibiotics may be ineffective.

Although penicillins are effective in treating many infections, they are sometimes overprescribed, so that resistant strains of bacteria develop, leading to "superinfections" that are difficult to cure. Resistance to antibiotics can also develop if you stop taking antibiotics as soon as the symptoms of an infection are gone. A few bacteria may survive with greater resistance, causing trouble later.

Penicillins are not the only antibiotics. The cephalosporins, for example, cefadroxil monohydrate (Duricef) and cefazolin sodium (Ancef), are used to treat serious infections, including septicemia (infection in the bloodstream) and bone and heart infections.

Tetracycline drugs are antibiotics used sometimes in mixed infections or when the infecting microbes cannot be identified.

Sulfonamides, or "sulfa" drugs, are effective in treating pneumonia, meningitis, and dysentery.

ANTIVIRAL DRUGS

Antibiotics do not work on viruses. Antiviral drugs work by becoming part of the virus in order to stop its ability to multiply. Examples of antiviral drugs are:

▲ Acyclovir (Zovirax), which is effective against herpes.

▲ AZT (Retrovir), which is used to treat HIV-positive and AIDS patients, especially those who have developed Pneumocystis pneumonia. Frequent blood tests are needed to monitor red blood cell counts since this drug can suppress their production in the bone marrow.

Another anti-infective drug is chloramphenicol, used to treat some forms of meningitis, salmonella, and other serious infections.

ANTIFUNGAL DRUGS

Besides bacteria and viruses, humans are subject to fungal infections. Fungi grow from tiny bodies called spores. They occur as superficial skin infections, yeast infections, rare and dangerous fevers, and some forms of meningitis. Fluconazole (Diflucan, Mycostatin, and others) is effective against fungal infections.

USING DRUGS WISELY

Never before in human history has there been such a vast array of potentially beneficial drugs available to treat illnesses as there is today. But their value depends greatly on how wisely they are prescribed by doctors and used by patients.

A detailed discussion of every existing drug and its side effects would require many volumes. At the end of this book, you will find a list of helpful guides to drugs for health care consumers. They are an invaluable aid to understanding your medication. In addition, your pharmacist can provide information about medications.

PART III
Next Steps

CHAPTER 11: ON LEAVING THE HOSPITAL:
No Place Like Home...............................114
Arranging for Home Care 114
Finding Support..115
Saying "Thanks"...115
Once You Are Home 115
Where to Get Information..116

On Leaving the Hospital:

NO PLACE LIKE HOME

Patients are now leaving the hospital soon after treatment. Ten years ago an appendectomy meant a five-day stay. Today, an uncomplicated appendectomy involves at most a two-day hospitalization. Most convalescing takes place at home and you may require some form of ongoing care. It is less costly to receive care at home than in the hospital and usually beneficial for you to be in a familiar environment over which you have some control.

ARRANGING FOR HOME CARE

Home care can take many forms. You may need physical therapy three times a week, a nurse to check your blood sugar or teach you how to do so, a home help aide to do light housekeeping, or any number of other services. Even if you need continuous intravenous therapy, you can be looked after at home, with daily visits from experienced nurses.

Arrangements for home care should be made before you leave the hospital. Make sure your doctor has given you instructions for ongoing care, including dates for follow-up appointments. You should get written instructions. Any prescriptions you may need can be filled by the hospital pharmacy or telephoned ahead to a pharmacy of your choice and picked up on the way home. If the medication is unfamiliar to you, ask the pharmacist for the patient information sheet about the drug.

Most hospitals have social workers, case managers, or discharge planners who are responsible for setting up home care. They can also arrange for any equipment you may need, such as crutches, wheelchairs, or even a hospital bed. They can set up transportation for continuing outpatient care, whether it's physical therapy, radiation treatments, chemotherapy, or dialysis. The National Association for Home Care is trying to get legislation that would require hospitals to provide discharged patients who may need home care with a list of providers in their area.

FINDING SUPPORT

If there are self-help or support groups related to your condition that you wish to contact, get their numbers before you leave the hospital. Such groups, for cancer survivors, people with heart problems, or parents of twins, to name just a few, can be beneficial. Social workers, pastoral care professionals, nurses, and doctors have such information. See "Where To Get Help" at the back of this book. If you feel you are being discharged from the hospital too soon, without a support network in place, speak to the administrative representative or clinical director who monitors length of stay. Those receiving Medicare can contact the local chapter of AARP or the Gray Panthers and ask to speak with the executive director for help in appealing a too-early discharge.

SAYING "THANKS"

If your hospital experience was positive, you can show your appreciation by writing to the administrator or sending cards, flowers, or candy to the staff on the unit where you were a patient. Some hospitals also have special award certificates that you can give to a particularly helpful employee. If your experience was bad, or you have questions, by all means contact the administration to complain or get more information. But make sure you have your facts straight, can document your experience, and understand that the hospital may have a different point of view

ONCE YOU ARE HOME

Prepare yourself to feel tired when you get home. Just stepping out into fresh air after even a couple of days in an enclosed hospital environment can be a shock to your system. Take a few deep breaths and don't try to do too much during the first few hours, days, or weeks. Take it easy. Your energy level may be low for a while.

If you have questions about your bill, be persistent. Complain if contacted inappropriately. One recently widowed woman's husband had died of cancer. Two weeks later she was briefly hospitalized for pneumonia. While recovering at home, she was cheerily telephoned with a reminder of her husband's next radiation treatment appointment. Obviously, they had failed to remove his name from their appointment list. The unwanted intrusion caused by a mistake like this underscores the need to protect yourself and those you care about from impersonal and unfeeling institutions.

WHERE TO GET INFORMATION

HOSPITALS

American Hospital Association
1 North Franklin Street
Chicago, IL 60606
(312) 422-3000
Has an annual *AHA Guide to the Health Care Field* with data on hospital accreditation.

Joint Commission on Accreditation
of Healthcare Organizations (JCAHO)
1 Renaissance Boulevard
Oak Brook Terrace, IL 60181
(708) 916-5600
Maintains list of accredited health care facilities and has a speakers' bureau.

DOCTORS

American Medical Association
Department of Physician Data Services
Dept. P, 515 N. State Street
Chicago, IL 60610
(312) 464-5000
Fax: (312) 464-4184
You can write for a profile of any member of the AMA; it keeps records on all doctors.

American Board of Medical Specialties
1007 Church Street, Suite 404
Evanston, IL 60201-5913
(708) 491-9091
Fax: (708) 328-3596
Concerned with maintenance of standards of doctors who are specialists; has database list and annual directory of certified medical specialists.

FOR OLDER HEALTH CONSUMERS

Medicare and Medicaid—
Department of Health and Human Services
1-800-638-6833 (Medicare Hotline)
Answers questions about Medicare.

Health Care Financing Administration (HCFA)
200 Independence Avenue SW, Room 314 G
Washington, DC 20201
(202) 690-6726
Fax: (202) 690-6262
Internet: http://www.ssa.gov/hcfa/hcfahp2.html
Oversees Medicare; can provide information on Medicare benefits.

American Association of Homes & Services for the Aging
901 E Street NW, Suite 500
Washington, DC 20004-2037
(202) 783-2242
Fax: (202) 783-2255
Members are voluntary, not-for-profit nursing homes, and retirement communities; it attempts to identify and solve problems with the help of Congress and federal agencies; provides publications.

American Health Care Association
1201 L Street NW
Washington, DC 20005
(202) 842-4444
Fax: (202) 842-3860
A federation of state associations of long-term care facilities, it promotes strategies for quality care; provides publications such as *Thinking About a Nursing Home?*

HEALTH MAINTENANCE ORGANIZATIONS (HMOS)

National Committee for Quality Assurance (NCQA)
2000 L Street NW, Suite 500
Washington, DC 20036
(202) 955-3500
Fax: (202) 955-3599
Ensures that each HMO's quality assurance program complies with national standards; conducts research, has training and education services, and a speakers' bureau.

Physicians Who Care
10615 Perrin Beitel Street, Suite 201
San Antonio, TX 78217
(210) 656-7636
1-800-545-9305
Fax: (210) 979-8235
A patient advocacy group devoted to maintaining the traditional doctor-patient relationship and ensuring quality health care; has publications and brochures.

MENTAL HEALTH

National Mental Health Association (NMHA)
1021 Prince Street
Alexandria, VA 22314-2971
(703) 684-7722 or 969-NMHA
Fax: (703) 684-5968
A consumer advocacy group that supports community mental health centers; visits facilities to assess care; is a central national source for educational material for the public.

The National Institute of Mental Health (NIMH)
5600 Fishers Lane, #7-99
Rockville, MD 20857
(301) 443-4513
Internet: nimhpubs@nih.gov
Researches the causes, diagnosis, treatment, and prevention of mental illness; provides information on mental health problems and programs.

National Mental Health Consumers' Self-Help Clearinghouse
1211 Chestnut Street
Philadelphia, PA 19107
(215) 751-1810
Fax: (215) 735-0275
Serves consumers and ex-patient self-help groups with information, referrals, technical help, and consulting for self-help programs; provides publications and a library open to the public.

SUPPORT GROUPS

National Health Information Center (NHIC)
P. O. Box 1133
Washington, DC 20013-1133
1-800-336-4797
(301) 565-4167
Fax: (301) 984-4256
Internet: nhicinfo@health.org or http://nhic-nt.health.org
A referral service to aid consumers; puts people with health questions in touch with organizations best able to provide answers; computer database of 1100 organizations (part of DIRLINE file of National Library of Medicine's MEDLARS).

National Cancer Institute, National Institutes of Health
Building 11, Room 10A24
Bethesda, MD 20892-3100
1-800-422-6273
(301) 496-5583
Conducts and funds research on cancer; sponsors regional and national cancer information services.

National Self-Help Clearinghouse
25 West 43rd Street
New York, NY 10036
(212) 354-8525
Helps people wishing to start a support group; refers to regional clearinghouses and support and self-help groups around the country.

Consumers' Union of the United States
101 Truman Avenue
Yonkers, NY 10703
(914) 378-2000
Gives information and advice on consumer goods and services that affect quality of life; regional offices represent consumers' interests in legislative agencies and the courts; publishes monthly *Consumer Reports* and other publications and studies.

Food and Drug Administration Office of Consumer Affairs
1-800-358-9295
(301) 443-3170
Fax: (301) 443-9767
Responsible for quality of drugs; investigates new drugs and problems with medications; responds to inquiries on issues; conducts consumer health education programs.

Public Citizen Health Research Group
2000 P Street NW, 7th Floor
Washington, DC 20036
(202) 833-3000
Fax: (202) 463-8842
Concerned with issues of health care delivery such as the safety of medical devices; petitions or sues federal agencies on consumers' behalf; publishes monthly *Health Letter* on health policy issues.

Bibliography

BOOKS ON DRUGS

Adderly, Brenda, ed. *The Complete Guide to Pills*. New York: Ballantine Books, 1997.

Brown, Ellen Hodgson, and Lynne Paige Walker. *The Informed Consumer's Pharmacy: The Essential Guide to Prescription and Over-the-Counter Drugs*. New York: Carroll and Graf, 1990.

Graedon, Joe, and Teresa Graedon, PhD. *The People's Pharmacy*. New York: St. Martin's Griffin, 1996.

Silverman, Harold M., Pharm.D. *The Pill Book*. New York: Bantam Books, 1996.

Winter, Ruth. *A Consumer's Dictionary of Medicines*. New York: Crown Trade Paperbacks, 1996.

CONSUMER HEALTH INFORMATION

Alpiar, Hal. *Doctor Shopping*. Bookworld, 1933 Whitfield Park Loop, Sarasota, FL 34243, 1996.

Consumers' Checkbook. *Consumers Guide to Hospitals*. 733 15th Street NW, Suite 820, Washington, DC 20005, (202) 347-7283

Consumers Union/Consumer Reports. *On Health* (monthly newsletter). P. O. Box 56356, Boulder, CO 80322. (513) 860-1178

Lesko, Matthew. *What to Do When You Can't Afford Health Care*. Info USA, P. O. Box 15700, Chevy Chase, MD 20815, 1993.

Miller, Marc S., ed. *Health Care Choices for Today's Consumer*. Living Planet Press, 2940 Newark Street NW, Washington, DC 20008, 1995.

Sribnick, Richard L., and Wayne B. Sribnick. *Smart Patient, Good Medicine: Working With Your Doctor to Get the Best Medical Care*. Walker and Co., 435 Hudson Street, New York, NY 10014, 1994.

Index

A

A-V node, 63
Acetaminophen, 108, 109
Acquired immune deficiency syndrome (AIDS), 70, 112
Acupuncture, 53
Acyclovir, 112
Adalat, 102
Administration. *see* Hospital administration
Adrenal glands, 69
Advance directive, 17, 18, 50-51
Aging, information resources about, 117
AIDS. *see* Acquired immune deficiency syndrome
Airway tubes, 83-84
Albuterol, 104
Ambien, 107
American Board of Surgery, 27
American Hospital Association, 25, 116
Aminophylline, 104
Amoxicillin, 111
Ampicillin, 111
Ancef, 111
Anesthesiologist
    choosing, 28 , nurse anesthetist, 38
Antacids, 105
Antianxiety drugs, 106-108
Antiarhythmics, 101-102
Antibiotics, 105, 111
Anticonvulsants, 108
Antifungal drugs, 112
Antihistamines, 104
Antihypertensives, 102
Antinausea drugs, 105
Antiulcer drugs, 105
Antiviral drugs, 112
Appendectomy, 10
Arrhythmia, 64
Arteriovenous shunt, 97
Arthritis, 67, 109
    rheumatoid, 67, 70
Aspirin, 103, 109
Asthma, 65
Atherosclerosis, 63
Ativan, 107
Atrovent, 104

Attending physicians. *see also* Doctors,
    at community hospitals, 10, 29
Attorney. *see also* Advance directive
    role in medical procedures, 26
Autoimmune diseases, 70. *see also* Immune system
AZT, 112

B

Baclofen, 106
Bactrim, 99
Barbituates, 107-108
Beds, 95, 114
Benadryl, 104
Benzodiazepines, 107
Billing. *see* Payments and fees
Bladder scanner, 90
Blood
    role in cardiovascular system, 62, 63,
    units of, 74
Blood banking, 59
Blood glucose monitoring, 96
Blood pressure cuff, 73-74
Blood tests
    choosing provider for, 30; for electrolyte levels and kidney functioning (BUN), 106; technicians for, 44-45
Blood thinners, 102-103
Blood transfusion, 74-75
Body systems. *see also specific body systems*
    cardiovascular system, 62-64; digestive system, 65; immune system, 70; metabolic system, 68-70; musculoskeletal system, 66-67; neurological system, 67-68; renal system, 66; respiratory system, 64-65
Bones, 66
Brain, 68
Brain tumor, 10
Bronchitis, 64
Bronchodilators, 104
Burn unit, 10
BuSpar, 107

C

Call button, 21
Carafate, 105
Carbamazepine, 108

Cardiopulmonary resuscitation (CPR), 50, 76
Cardiovascular system
    blood, 64; heart, 63;
    medical equipment and procedures, 71-72
        blood pressure cuff/stethoscope, 73-74;
        blood transfusion, 74-75; central line,
        75-76, crash cart, 76-77; defibrillators,
        77; electrocardiogram, 78; implanted
        catheter, 78; intravenous lines, 44-45, 78-
        80, 82-83; IV pumps, 80; needles and
        syringes, 81-82; saline locks, 82; teleme-
        try, 83;
    medications
        antiarrhythmics, 101-102
        antihypertensives, 102; blood thinners,
        102-103; cholesterol-lowering drugs,
        103; digoxin, 99, 103, 106; nitroglycerin,
        103-104; problems with, 63-64
Cardizem, 102
Care, acute vs. chronic, 10
Case managers. *see* Social workers
Casts, 93
CAT. *see* Computerized axial tomography
Catapres, 102
Catheters
    Foley catheter, 90-91; "in and out," 90-91
CBI. *see* Continuous bladder irrigation
Central line, 75-76
Cephalosporins, 111
Change-of-shift report, 20
Chest tubes, 84
Chief Executive Officer (CEO). *see* Hospital
    administration
Children, visiting policies for, 52
Chlordiazepoxide, 107
Cholesterol-lowering drugs, 103
Clerks, 44
Clinical clerks, 29
Clonazepam, 107, 108
Cloxacillin, 111
"Code blue," 76
Code of Patients Rights. *see* Patients Bill of Rights
Colds, 64
Colostomies, 89-90, 92
Community hospitals, 10, 11, 29
Complaints, 24, 32, 56, 115. *see also* Legal disputes
Computerized axial tomography (CAT) scan, 45
Consent forms, 14, 29
Consumer information, resources for, 120
Continuous bladder irrigation (CBI), 91-92
Continuous positive airway pressure (CPAP), 85
Corticosteroids, 109, 110
"Cost review" companies, 26
Coumadin, 103
CPAP. *see* Continuous positive airway pressure
CPR. *see* Cardiopulmonary resuscitation
Crash cart, 76-77
Credentials committee, 24
Crutches, 95, 114
Cystostomy tube, 92

D

Dalmane, 107
Darvocet, 108
Darvon, 108
Decadron, 109
Defibrillators, 77
Deltasone, 110
Dementia, 39, 107
Demerol, 108
Depakane, 108
DiaBeta, 110
Diabetes, 69, 96
    drugs for, 109-110
Diagnostic Related Groupings (DRGs), 12
Dialysis, 97, 115. *see also* Renal system
Diazepam, 107
Dietician, 46
Digestive system
    gallbladder, 65; liver, 65; medical equipment
    and procedures, 72; colostomies, 89-90, 92;
    feeding tubes, 87-88; nasogastric (NG) tubes,
    88-89; total parenteral nutrition (TPN), 89
    medications
        antacids, 105; antinausea drugs, 105;
        antiulcer drugs, 105
    pancreas, 65; problems with, 65
Digoxin, 99, 103, 106
Dilantin, 108
Dilaudid, 108
Diuretics, 102, 105-106
DNR. *see* "Do Not Resuscitate"
"Do Not Resuscitate" (DNR) order, 50, 76
Dobbhoff tube, 87
Doctors. *see also* Specialists
    at community hospitals, 10, 29; choosing,
    27-28; communicating with, 27, 28-29, 33-
    34; foreign-trained, 33; getting information
    about, 116-117; hospital supervision of, 32-
    33; interns, 30; medical audit review of, 24-
    25; qualities of, 27, 33-34; residents, 29,
    30-31; types of, 34
Dopamine, 68
"Dr. Leo" code, 76
Drains, 93
Dramamine, 105
DRGs. *see* Diagnostic Related Groupings
Drugs. *see* Medications
Duricef, 111
Dysentery, 111

E

Echocardiogram, 45
Edema, 105
EKG. *see* Electrocardiogram
EKG technicians, duties of, 45
Electrocardiogram (EKG), 45, 63, 78
Emergencies, coded announcements for, 76
Emergency room (ER), 13
Emphysema, 64-65

Encephalitis, 68
Endocrine system, 68, 69
Endotracheal tube, 83
Epilepsy, 68, 108
Epinephrine, 102, 104
Epogen, 106
ER. *see* Emergency room
Erythromycin, 111
Erythropoietin, 106
Ethical considerations, 21-22, 31, 32, 42
Exocrine system, 69

F

Family. *see also* Visiting; Visitors
    accommodations for, 19, 47, 51-52; com-
    plaints by, 24; support groups for, 48
Feeding tubes, 87-88
Fluconazole, 112
Food, choices for, 19, 53
Fosamax, 106
Friends. *see also* Visitors
    good qualities for, 54-55
Furosemide, 105-106

G

Gallbladder, 65
Gallbladder surgery, 10
Gifts, for hospital staff, 42, 115
Glucotrol, 110
Gout, 67, 109

H

Halcion, 107
Halos and tongs, 94
HCFA. *see* Health Care Financing Administration
Health Care Financing Administration (HCFA),
    12, 58, 117
Health educators, duties of, 46
Health Maintenance Organizations (HMOs), 58
    getting information about, 118; hospital
    choices with, 15; physician choices with, 27-28
Heart, 62, 63
Heart attack, 63-64, 102
Heart failure, congestive, 64, 99, 103
Heart function, tests for determining, 45
Hemodialysis, 97
Heparin, 81, 102
Hip replacement, 10, 67
HIV. *see* Human immunodeficiency virus
HMOs. *see* Health Maintenance Organizations
Holistic therapies, 52-53
Holter monitor, 45, 83
Home care, arranging for, 114-115
Hospital administration
    administrator's responsibilities, 23-24; qual-
    ity assurance responsibilities, 24-25
Hospital admissions
    admission process, 15-17; choosing a hospital,
    13-14; elective, 13, 15; emergency (ER), 13;
    questions to ask, 14, 59; uninsured procedure,

17; VIP treatment, 21-22; what to bring with
    you, 16
Hospital amenities
    food, 19; Patients' Bill of Rights, 18; rooms,
    12, 17, 19, 51
Hospital costs, discussed, 12
Hospital discharge, 21, 59, 115
Hospital inspections, 11-12
Hospital room
    amenities of, 17; charges and costs for, 12, 59,
    60; private vs. semiprivate, 17, 56; visiting in,
    19, 51-52
Hospital workers. *see also* Doctors; Nurses
    clerks, 44; EKG technicians, 45; food services
    staff, 49; health educators, 46; imaging tech-
    nicians, 45; infection control, 46; laboratory
    technicians, 44-45; mental health staff, 48;
    pastoral care staff, 47; patient representatives,
    48; pharmacy staff, 45; porters, 49; rehabilita-
    tion specialists, 46-47; social workers, 47;
    volunteers, 49
Hospitals
    financing mechanisms, 9, 24; getting infor-
    mation about, 116; state-run, 33;
    structure of, 19-21
        nurses, 19; staffing levels, 20, 32, 41-42;
        unit clerk, 20; supervision of physicians,
        32-33
    types of, 9-11;
        community hospitals, 10, 11; government
        hospitals, 11; specialty hospitals, 11;
        teaching hospitals, 10
Housing, for family, 19, 47
Human immunodeficiency virus (HIV), 70, 112

I

Ibuprofen, 109
ID badges, 39, 44, 49
Ileal conduits, 92
Imaging technicians, 47
Immune system
    disorders of, 70; drugs for, 110-111
Implanted catheter, 78
Incentive spirometer, 84
Inderal, 102
Infection
    bacterial/viral, 64; body response to, 63, 70
Infection control, 46
Infertility clinic, 10
Inflammation, of blood vessels, 64
Injections. *see also* Intravenous lines
    intradermal, 81; intramuscular (IM), 81;
    subcutaneous (SQ), 81
Insulin, 69, 81, 96, 109
    types of, 110
Insurance. *see also* Payments and fees
    administration procedures, 23; costs and
    schedules, 12, 60; discharge requirements, 21;
    hospital eligibility for, 13-14; preauthoriza-
    tion process, 15, 59

Intravenous lines. *see also* Injections
    choosing provider for, 30-31; home process for,
    114; implanted, 78-80; "IV Team," 44-45; pro-
    cedures for starting, 74-75; secondary, 82-83
Invasive procedures, choosing provider for, 30

J
JCAHO. *see* Joint Commission on Accreditation
    of Healthcare Organizations
Joint Commission on Accreditation of Health-
    care Organizations (JCAHO), 11, 116
Joints, 67
Jordan, Claire, 42
Journal writing, 53

K
Kidney stones, 93
Kidneys
    role in renal system, 66; tests for, 106
Klonopin, 107, 108
Knee replacement, 67

L
Laboratory technicians, 44-45
Lanoxin, 99
Laryngoscope, 83
Lasix, 105
Legal disputes. *see also* Complaints
    mediation of, 48; value of records in, 26
Librium, 107
Lifestyle issues, 43
Lioresal, 106
Liver, 65
Lopressor, 102
Lorazepam, 107
Lortab, 108
Lovastatin, 103
Lovenox, 103
Lumbar puncture, 30, 96
Lungs, 64
Lupus, 70
Lymphocytic immune globulin, 111

M
Maalox, 105
Magnetic resonance imaging (MRI) scan, 45
Maintenance, 20, 23
Malpractice litigation, 32-33
Managed care programs, 42, 58
    hospital choices with, 13, 15; physician
    choices with, 27
Marinol, 105
Massage, 52
Medicaid, 58
    getting information about, 117
Medical audit committee, 24-25
Medical equipment and procedures
    for cardiovascular system, 71-72; for digestive
    system, 72, 87-90; for musculoskeletal system,
    72-73, 93-95; for neurological system, 73, 96;

for pain control, 73, 97-98; for renal system,
    72, 90-93; for respiratory system, 72, 83-87
Medical information. *see also* Questions
    sources for obtaining, 28
Medical records
    confidentiality of, 18; discharge summary,
    26; keeping copies of, 25-26
"Medical review" companies, 26
Medical students, role in teaching hospital, 29-30
Medicare
    costs and fees, 12, 13, 57, 58, 115; discharge re-
    quirements, 21; getting information about, 117
Medications
    antibiotics, 105, 111; antifungal drugs, 112;
    antiviral drugs, 112; billed in error, 59; for
    cardiovascular system, 101-104; "controlled"
    drugs, 100; delivery and administration of,
    100-101; for digestive system, 105; drug
    interactions, 101; generic and brand name
    drugs, 99; hospital "formulary," 45, 100; hos-
    pital prescription for, 99-100; IV delivery of,
    79; for metabolic system, 109-110; for mus-
    culoskeletal system, 106; for neurological sys-
    tem, 106-109; nurses responsibility for,
    36-37, 40-41, 99-100; prescription, 16, 55,
    100, 114; PRN medications, 41; for renal sys-
    tem, 105-106; for respiratory system, 104;
    tips for appropriate use, 101
Medicolegal committee, 25
Meditation, 52, 53
Meningitis, 68, 107, 111
Mental health staff, 48
Mental illness, 33, 39
    getting information about, 118-119
Metabolic system, 68-69
    adrenal glands, 69
    medical equipment and procedures
        blood glucose monitoring, 96; dialysis, 97
    medications
        corticosteroids, 109, 110; diabetes drugs,
        109-110; for immune system, 110-111;
        thyroid medication, 110
    pancreas, 69, 96; pituitary gland, 69; thyroid
        gland, 69
Metoprolol, 102
MI. *see* Myocardial infarction
Morphine, 108
Mortality and morbidity committee, 25
Motrin, 109
MRI. *see* Magnetic resonance imaging
Multiple sclerosis, 67, 106, 109
Muscles, tendons, ligaments, 66
Musculoskeletal system
    bones, 66; joints, 67
    medical equipment and procedures, 72-73
        casts/traction, 93; drains, 93; halos and
        tongs, 94; restraints, 94; sutures and sta-
        ples, 95; wheelchairs and devices, 95
    medications, 106; muscles, tendons, ligaments,
    66; problems with, 67

Mylanta, 105
Myocardial infarction (MI), 64

N

Narcotics, 108
Nasogastric (NG) tubes, 88-89
National Association for Home Care, 115
Needles and syringes, 81-82
Nembutal, 107
Nephrostomy tube, 92
Nerves, 67-68
Nervous system, sympathetic/parasympathetic, 68
Neurological system
  brain, 68
  medical equipment and procedures, 73
    lumbar puncture, 96
  medications
    antianxiety drugs, 106-108; anticonvulsants, 108; narcotics, 108; pain medications, 108-109
  nerves, 67-68; nervous system, 68
Nifedipine, 102
Nitroglycerin, 103-104
Nosocomial infection, 46
Nuclear medicine, 45
Nurses. *see also* Hospital workers
  charge nurse, 19, 20, 49, 56; dress codes, 39; gifts to, 42, 115
  in hospital structure, 19-21
    certified nursing assistant (CNA), 38; licensed practical nurse (LPN), 37; licensed vocational nurse (LVN), 37; registered nurses (RN), 37
  private-duty, 42; procedures of, 36-37; qualities of, 43; referrals to doctors from, 28
  responsibilities of
    at each shift, 40; care and medications, 36-37, 40-41, 115; paperwork, 41
  specialty
    certified nurse midwife (CNM), 38; clinical nurse specialist (CNS), 38; "community liaison," 58; nurse anesthetist, 38; nurse clinician (NC), 46; nurse practitioner (NP), 38
  staffing pattern, 20, 41-42, 56; and unit clerk, 20; and unlicensed staff, 42
Nursing home placement, 47

O

Occupational therapy (OT), 47
Ombudsman. *see* Patient representative
Ondansetron, 105
Orthopedic technology, 47
Osteoarthritis, 67
Osteoporosis, 67
Ostomies, 92
OT. *see* Occupational therapy
Oxazepam, 107
Oxygen
  continuous positive airway pressure (CPAP), 85; and oxygen therapy, 84-85

P

Pain. *see also* Medications
  medications for, 41, 108-109
Pain control
  medical equipment and procedures, 73
  patient-controlled anesthesia (PCA), 97-98 ;
  transcutaneous electrical nerve stimulation (TENS), 98
Pancreas
  role in digestive system, 65; role in metabolic system, 69, 96
Parkinson's disease, 68
Pastoral care staff, 47, 115
Patient
  communicating with physician, 28-29; as "good" or "poor" historian, 29; relation with nurses, 20, 39, 40, 43, 53, 56; 10 tips for, 55-56
Patient accounts office, 60
Patient needs, 40, 53-54
Patient records. *see* Medical records
Patient representative
  duties and responsibilities of, 48; nurses' role as, 37, 43; obtaining records from, 26
Patient-controlled anesthesia (PCA), 97-98
Patients' Bill of Rights, 14, 17, 25
  discussed, 18
Patients' issues
  advance directive, 17, 18, 50-51; holistic therapies, 52-53; qualities of good patient, 53-54; visiting policies, 51-52
Payments and fees. *see also* Insurance
  cost reduction strategies, 59-60; errors in, 59; hospital billing practices, 58-59; Medicare, 12, 13, 57; questions about, 116; "scholarship" patients, 12, 57-58; for uninsured patient, 60
PCA. *see* Patient-controlled anesthesia
PEG tube. *see* Percutaneous endoscopic gastrostomy tube
Penicillin, 111
Pentobarbital, 107
Percocet, 108
Percutaneous endoscopic gastrostomy (PEG) tube, 87-88
Peritoneal dialysis, 97
Pharmacy. *see also* Medications
  staff and "formulary," 45, 100
Phenergan, 105
Phenytoin, 108
Physical therapy (PT), 46-47
  after stroke, 10
Physicians. *see* Doctors; Specialists
Pituitary gland, 69
Pneumonia, 64, 70, 84, 111
Polyps, 65
Posey vest, 94
Power of attorney. *see also* Advance directive
  procedures for, 50-51
PPOs. *see* Preferred Provider Organizations
Pranic healing, 52-53

Prayer, 53
Prednisone, 109, 110
Preferred Provider Organizations (PPOs), 15
Primary nursing. *see also* Nurses
staffing approach, 20
Privacy concerns, 18, 49
Procardia, 102
Proventil, 104
Psychiatrists, 33, 35, 48. *see also* Specialists
Psychologists, 48
PT. *see* Physical therapy
Public relations, 23, 24
Pulse oximetry, 85

Q

Quality assurance, administrators' responsibilities for, 24-25
Questions
about your bill, 116; to ask at admission, 14; to ask your doctor, 28-29, 33; to ask your nurse, 40, 43; patient's and visitor's responsibilities for, 42, 54, 56
Quinidine, 102

R

Radiology, 30, 31, 45
Recreational therapy, 47
Regulations, 24
Rehabilitation facility placement, 47, 58
Rehabilitation specialists, 46-47
Renal system
kidneys, 66
medical equipment and procedures, 72
bladder scanner, 90; catheters, 90-91; continuous bladder irrigation (CBI), 91-92; ostomies, 92; urine collectors, 92-93
medications, diuretics, 102, 105-106; problems with, 66
Research studies, 18
Respiratory system
lungs, 64
medical equipment and procedures, 72, 83-87
airway tubes, 83-84; chest tubes, 84; incentive spirometer, 84; oxygen, 84-85; pulse oximetry, 85; suction machine, 85; tracheostomy, 86; ventilators, 86-87
medications
antihistamines, 104; bronchodilators, 104; epinephrine, 104
problems with, 64-65
Respiratory therapy (RT), 46
Restoril, 107
Restraints, 94
Retrovir, 112
Rheumatoid arthritis, 67, 70
Risk management, 25
Ronald McDonald houses, 19
RT. *see* Respiratory therapy

S

Salaries
nurses, 37; resident physician, 30
Schizophrenia, 68
"Scholarship patients," 12, 57-58
Seconal, 107
Second opinions, 26, 28, 34
Self-hypnosis, 52
Septicemia, 111
Septra, 99
Serax, 107
Sleep apnea, 85
Sliding boards, 95
Social workers, 47, 115
Specialists. *see also* Doctors
at teaching hospital, 29, 30, 31; choosing, 14, 27; nurses, 38; types of, 35
Speech therapy, 46
Spinal tap, 30, 96
Steri strips, 95
Stethoscope, 73-74
Stoma, 92
Streptokinase, 102
Stress
affecting nurses, 41-42, 43; reducing with information, 22
Stroke, 10, 48, 64, 88, 103
Substance abuse, 43, 48
Suction machine, 85
Sulfonamides, 111
Support groups, 48
getting information about, 119; for home care, 115
Support persons, good qualities for, 54-55
Suprapubic catheter, 92
Surgery
outpatient or day-surgery basis, 15; performed by specialist, 31
Sutures and staples, 95
Synthroid, 110

T

Tachycardia, 103
Talwin, 108
TCM. *see* Traditional Chinese medicine
Teaching hospital
advantages of, 32; characteristics of, 10
hierarchy
medical students, 29-30; residents, 30-31, 32; specialists, 31
Team approach, for nurse staffing, 20
Tegretol, 108
Telemetry, 83
Television, 56
Temazepam, 107
TENS. *see* Transcutaneous electrical nerve stimulation
Tests
arranging for, 55, 59; errors in, 60

Tetracycline drugs, 111
Tetrahydrocannabinol, 105
Texas Nurses Association, 42
Theft, protection against, 16, 55
Theophylline, 104
"Three strikes, you're out" rule, 31
Thyroid gland, role in metabolic system, 69
Tissue committee, 24
Total parenteral nutrition (TPN), 89
TPN. *see* Total parenteral nutrition
Tracheostomy, 86
Traction
    skeletal, 93; skin, 93
Traditional Chinese medicine (TCM), 53
Transcutaneous electrical nerve stimulation
    (TENS), 98
Treadmill test, 45
Triage, 13
Triazolam, 107
Tylenol, 108, 109

U

Unlicensed staff, and nurses, 42
Ureterostomies, 92
Urethra, 66

Urine, 66, 90. *see also* Renal system
Utilization review department, 24

V

Vaccines, 111
Valium, 107
Vancomycin, 111
Ventilators, 86-87
Verapamil, 102
VIP treatment, 21-22
Visiting hours, 19
Visiting policies, 51-52
Visitors, good qualities for, 54-55
Visualization techniques, 52

W

Walkers, 95
Wheelchairs, 95, 114

X

X-ray records, 26

Z

Zovirax, 112

Other books in the Vital Information Series

Perimenopause
By Bernard Cortese, M.D.

Perimenopause describes the changes that may take place during the transitional time before and after menopause, discusses the pros and cons of hormone replacement therapy (HRT), offers alternative treatments. A practical guide.

$11.95 • ISBN 0-89594-914-8

Surgery
By Molly Shapiro, M.B.A., R.N.

Surgery covers every aspect of the surgery process including what your rights are as a patient. It tells you how to prepare for surgery, what happens in surgery, explains equipment use and procedures, and addresses your post-op concerns.

$11.95 • ISBN 0-89594-898-2

Vitamins, Minerals & Supplements
By Gayle Skowronski and Beth Petro Roybal

Vitamins, Minerals & Supplements gives information about the role of supplements in nutrition and how to choose them wisely. It gives details for specific common nutritional supplements and the daily requirements necessary for good health.

$11.95 • ISBN 0-89594-935-0

To receive a current catalog from The Crossing Press,
please call toll-free, 800-777-1048.
Visit our Website on the Internet at: www.crossingpress.com